T0219981

Tackling Health Anxiety:
A CBT Handbook

Tackling Health Anxiety: A CBT Handbook

Helen Tyrer

RCPsych Publications

CAMBRIDGE
UNIVERSITY PRESS

University Printing House, Cambridge CB2 8BS, United Kingdom

One Liberty Plaza, 20th Floor, New York, NY 10006, USA

477 Williamstown Road, Port Melbourne, VIC 3207, Australia

314-321, 3rd Floor, Plot 3, Splendor Forum, Jasola District Centre, New Delhi - 110025, India

103 Penang Road, #05-06/07, Visioncrest Commercial, Singapore 238467

Cambridge University Press is part of the University of Cambridge.

It furthers the University's mission by disseminating knowledge in the pursuit of education, learning and research at the highest international levels of excellence.

www.cambridge.org
Information on this title: www.cambridge.org/9781908020901

© The Royal College of Psychiatrists 2013

RCPsych Publications is an imprint of the Royal College of Psychiatrists,
17 Belgrave Square, London SW1X 8PG
http://www.rcpsych.ac.uk

A catalogue record for this publication is available from the British Library

ISBN 978-1-908-02090-1 Paperback

Distributed in North America by Publishers Storage and Shipping Company.

For Paula and Rick

Contents

List of tables, boxes, figures and case examples

Foreword

I am very pleased to recommend this book by Dr Tyrer to assist the training of a wide range of professionals working in healthcare. We think we know a great deal about illness in hospitals, but we tend to forget that a large part of it has a psychological component. What surprised me after reading this book was how common health anxiety is in medical clinics. If one in five people has the condition, it must lead to a great deal of suffering. I also note with some pleasure that the modification of cognitive–behavioural therapy developed by Dr Tyrer is especially suited to nurses working in general hospitals. Nurses are in a unique position here; they understand the medical problems of the people they are caring for and, after reading this book and receiving what I hope will be further training locally, they will then be able to understand the additional problems that are a direct consequence of health anxiety. Other professionals such as psychologists and psychiatrists may be equally competent in giving this treatment, but often will not give the same level of confidence that a well-trained nurse will give in administering this therapy.

I also like the balance of theory and practice in this book. We not only need to understand the principles behind treatment, but also have a good idea of what happens in practice. The case examples described by Dr Tyrer ring true and I am sure they will be of great value to practitioners when they are trying to disentangle psychological from physical problems in the patients that they see. I also hope that this book adds to the growing understanding that when patients present to any part of the National Health Service they should receive a full assessment of both their psychological and physical status; for rather too long, the psychological aspects have been ignored.

Dr Peter Carter
Chief Executive and General Secretary
Royal College of Nursing

Preface

I have written this book to help health professionals in their management of people who used to be diagnosed with hypochondria, but whom I think are better described as having health anxiety. I work mainly in general hospital settings and we now know that somewhere between 10 and 20% of all patients attending clinics in general hospitals have pathological health anxiety. It is pathological because it creates enormous suffering and disability and this often goes on for years in the absence of treatment. At present it is unfortunate that most of these people continue to attend clinics in search of a treatment not for their anxiety, but for the disease or diseases that they suspect they might have.

Although there are psychological services for people with health anxiety, only a small proportion of those with the condition are ever seen. This is partly because it is so common, partly because many people feel stigmatised by the suggestion that they might need psychological input for what they suspect is a physical condition, and partly because those who already have a physical disorder but also have abnormal health anxiety are not normally seen by the psychology services. I believe fervently that the best way of managing health anxiety successfully and economically is for front-line staff in medical services to both recognise and treat these patients in the clinics where they present repeatedly. They should be treated by staff who are part of the general services, not referred to a specialised clinic. So general and specialised nurses of all grades, occupational therapists, physiotherapists, dietitians, and support staff with relatively little in the way of formal qualifications, as well as psychologists, can all become competent in both identifying people with health anxiety and giving them advice and treatment. This is not a belief; it has recently been reinforced by evidence from a large randomised trial (Tyrer *et al*, 2013).

What I hope is that the necessary advice and treatment is given in this book. It is all based on my practice over the past 12 years and work in developing this treatment, and I am indebted to Professor Paul Salkovskis in first showing me the essentials of this important modification of cognitive–behavioural therapy (CBT) that lie at the heart of management.

In my work I have been helped greatly by my patients in developing this treatment further in all branches of medicine. I have therefore concentrated on giving practical examples of treatment, including case examples, all of which are fictitious in that they do not identify people, but accurate in that they describe problems that have arisen in therapy and how they can be overcome.

We are a long way off from what I would like to see as the comprehensive assessment of all patients when they first present at hospital clinics, when the accuracy and expertise of the medical assessment is matched equally by the quality and sophistication of the psychological one, but I hope that the proper assessment of health anxiety can be incorporated into this ideal scenario soon. This book is a start.

I thank John Rowley and Nick Wight especially for their encouragement in allowing me to develop this work, Elizabeth Carlin and the staff of the genitourinary medicine department at Kings Mill Hospital for starting me off on this journey, and my husband, Peter, for his constant support.

H.T.

Part I

Principles and practice of CBT for health anxiety

CHAPTER 1

Introduction

Excessive, or abnormal, health anxiety is a form of anxiety focused on the belief of having, or fear of getting, a serious illness. The belief or fear is usually concerned with a medical illness and occurs without sufficient evidence of organic pathology to account for the symptoms, and despite medical reassurance. Both health anxiety and organic illness can coexist. For diagnostic purposes, health anxiety is normally not regarded as pathological until it has lasted for at least 6 months.

Worrying about health is a normal protective function. For example, in someone with a history of chest pain due to angina, the natural concern arising from more frequent attacks may prompt a medical consultation which could avert an impending myocardial infarction. Health anxiety becomes maladaptive when it is out of proportion to the medical risk. This could represent either a low level of anxiety when the risk is high, as, for example, indulging in frequent episodes of unprotected sex with many partners, with little or no consideration of the risk of acquiring a sexually transmitted infection, or experiencing excessive worry about a potential medical problem when in fact the risk of developing that condition is normal or very low.

Severity may range from mild concern to severe and constant preoccupation. The problem may also be transient; from time to time we all experience health anxiety which subsequently resolves, but for some it may become chronic and debilitating and cause severe suffering, which unfortunately in many cases becomes persistent.

The term 'health anxiety' is increasingly being used to describe patients with hypochondriasis. Its main advantage over hypochondriasis is that as well as being more accurate, it is less pejorative and therefore more acceptable to patients and makes it easier to broach the diagnosis. It is used throughout the text in this handbook, and is likely to become a formal diagnosis in the near future. In patients with this condition, preoccupation with health arising from cognitions based on the misinterpretations of bodily sensations and changes, generates a range of distressing emotions. Interpreting everything in the worst way (catastrophic thinking) and the associated images of the terrible consequences of developing the feared disease often lead to severe disability.

Patients with health anxiety may express fear of developing a disease in the future, despite being free of symptoms at the time. More usually, they misinterpret symptoms and bodily sensations as evidence of severe underlying disease. Some experience long-standing symptoms or sensations (often medically unexplained), which they are convinced represent severe underlying disease. There are also those with the diagnosis who have proven physical disease but have health concerns with regard to fears and symptoms that are disproportionate to their underlying condition.

Prevalence

The prevalence of a disorder refers to the proportion of a particular population affected by a condition at any one time. There is a wide variation in the estimation of the prevalence of health anxiety within different medical settings, with figures for primary care ranging from 0.8% (Gureje *et al*, 1997) to 4.5% (Faravelli *et al*, 1997). Studies of more specialist populations have tended to show higher prevalence rates, with Aydemir and colleagues (1997) showing a point prevalence rate among cardiology patients with permanent pacemakers of 7.4%. However, a recent large-scale study using a standardised questionnaire, the Health Anxiety Inventory (HAI; Salkovskis *et al*, 2002), in nearly 30 000 medical patients showed a rate of 19.8% (Tyrer *et al*, 2011a). This may represent a slight overestimate, as many patients with medical conditions requiring close monitoring may have excessive health anxiety that is to some extent justified, but it nonetheless illustrates we are dealing with a very common condition.

The prevalence rates in psychiatric populations, including patients seen in liaison psychiatry with chronic pain, have showed higher prevalence levels at 10–15%, but the methods of assessment have varied greatly (Polatin *et al*, 1993; Altamura *et al*, 1998; Gatchel *et al*, 2006). The prevalence rates reported in secondary care are also higher, but a great deal depends on the degree to which the populations are selected or unselected. If unselected, the rates are lower – Barsky *et al* (1990) found the 6-month prevalence of DSM-III-R hypochondriasis to be only between 4.2 and 6.3% of consecutive attenders at a medical clinic.

Prevalence rates also tend to be understandably higher when populations of patients with medically unexplained symptoms are studied, as individuals with health anxiety as well as other pathology are included. Nimnuan *et al* (2001) found in a survey of seven general medical clinics that no less than 52% of the patients had medically unexplained symptoms, the highest proportion in gynaecological clinics. It is likely that a significant proportion of these patients, at least 40%, would have health anxiety too.

In a more recent study we found the prevalence of significant health anxiety in genitourinary medicine clinics to be between 8.6 and 10.2%

(Seivewright *et al*, 2004), and a similar study conducted in medical out-patients suggests the prevalence is between 12 and 15%, and even higher (up to 25%) in neurology clinics (Tyrer *et al*, 2011a).

Overlap with medically unexplained symptoms

Many cases of health anxiety may be missed, at least initially, when patients present to medical services, partly because of overlap with medically unexplained symptoms. The concern expressed by the patient and the nature of their symptoms may readily prompt investigation or further referral. These may be justified initially but, typically, it is only after these, often extensive, investigations have run their course and no pathology has been found that the problem is seen exactly for what it is, a non-disease.

There is often a discrepancy between the severity of symptoms and their underlying pathology. Ruo *et al* (2003), in a study of patients with chronic cardiac disease, found little association between severity of symptoms and the degree of underlying pathology. Of course, a medical explanation is not always available for every bodily sensation or change. Some patients, particularly those who like to have an answer to everything, find this concept difficult to accept, saying things such as, 'My doctor has told me what *is not* wrong with me, but he hasn't said what is causing the discomfort'. This uncertainty can be difficult for some to accept, leading to continuing attendance in primary care, and accounting for up to a half of all out-patient consultations (Nimnuan *et al*, 2001). Together, this constitutes a considerable burden of care, especially as there is no evidence in these cases that hunting for hidden underlying organic pathology is likely to reveal a cause.

Historically, medically unexplained symptoms have been considered as evidence of 'hidden' psychopathology. Too painful to be acknowledged in terms of psychological distress, they have somehow become 'somatised' into physical, and hence possibly more acceptable, phenomena. Although this theory remains in the popular domain, there is absolutely no evidence to support it (Mayou *et al*, 2005).

In some cases where patients experience many symptoms they may be given a diagnosis of a functional somatic syndrome. Not all patients given such diagnoses have high health anxiety, but a proportion will, although we do not know how many. These diagnoses, including irritable bowel syndrome (IBS), fibromyalgia, unexplained vomiting syndrome and chronic fatigue syndrome, are given by the physician to attempt to explain or 'label' otherwise unexplained symptoms in the particular specialty concerned. This rarely serves the patient well. These conditions have poor outcomes, and giving an organic label, rather than that of medically unexplained symptoms, makes it harder to manage them and address any underlying psychopathology. Many such patients use health services frequently (Lloyd & Pender, 1992; Bombardier & Buchwald, 1996; Kroenke *et al*, 1997; Barsky *et al*, 2005). Not all these patients will access mainstream services; many will search out alternative treatments, sometimes incurring large expense, with some abandoning hope of ever finding a cure or symptomatic relief. It is uncertain how many of these patients have health anxiety, but many during the course of their illness will qualify for more than one functional disorder. Identifying related anxiety in these patients and addressing it with cognitive–behavioural therapy (CBT) can produce considerable relief and prevent a great deal of suffering. It also facilitates medical management.

Giving a likely diagnosis of medically unexplained symptoms and discussion with the patient of how commonly this condition occurs in medical settings, can help make sense of what is occurring and lead to a more appropriate style of management. However, it is impossible to say that any symptom presenting is unequivocally psychological in origin before medical assessment has been completed.

In the face of this dilemma, where symptoms are troublesome and frequently failing to fit in with normal medical expectations, we need a new solution. We are now beginning to move towards a more comprehensive multidisciplinary approach. This approach considers the contribution of social, psychological and biological factors to all aspects of the condition and so avoids traditional separation of patients into having either a medical problem or a psychiatric one.

Why health anxiety is important

Health anxiety is common and underdiagnosed in medical settings. It causes considerable morbidity, tends to persist without specific intervention, and generates significant cost (Barsky *et al*, 2005; Seivewright *et al*, 2008). Costs are incurred because of more frequent medical consultations, more unnecessary and frequently expensive investigations, more referrals to other specialties, and frequent attendances at emergency care facilities, leading to unnecessary hospital admissions. Many of the more complex investigations also carry additional risk. Failure to address health anxiety properly can also lead to a breakdown in the relationship between the patient and health professionals, leading to complaints and further compromising care.

Health anxiety with pre-existing physical disease

Pathological health anxiety can be present in those with established physical disease, and this often complicates management. Coexistence with other disease (often called comorbidity) is not a bar to treatment with therapies such as CBT, and successful management of these patients can greatly improve their quality of life. This comorbidity is discussed in more detail in Part 2, but examples include recurrent non-cardiac chest pain following a myocardial infarction, anxiety-related irritable bowel syndrome complicating Crohn's disease and excessive breathlessness and panic in chronic obstructive pulmonary disease.

Rationale for providing psychological treatment within medical settings

For patients who already have established physical disease it seems particularly relevant to address their fears within a medical setting. Indeed, in cardiology services many patients already progress to cardiac rehabilitation where they receive graded, supervised exercise regimes, education and relaxation training from members of the team, which have a strong psychological component. It would be ideal if these same people could receive CBT when necessary within the same framework, delivered by the specially trained staff who have understanding of their medical problems. This approach expands the role of all health professionals beyond the immediate needs of physical and lifestyle management, and represents not only a more sophisticated, but a more sensible model of care.

Currently, patients who are identified in medical settings as experiencing obvious psychological problems are either referred back to their general practitioner (GP), if there is no need for continued medical care in the clinic, or referred elsewhere for a psychological assessment. What often happens is that their medical care may continue without any specific effort to address health anxiety apart from reassurance, so often shown in the form of more frequent, but medically pointless, follow-up.

There is often a significant wait for psychological assessment and after the referral has been made, it is common for patients to be invited to 'opt in' to the service. Health-anxious patients, who often resent referral to a psychologist, believing that the doctor now assumes their problem is 'all in the mind', remain convinced that there is something physically wrong that requires further investigation. They often fail to attend their psychological assessment, or decline to opt in to demonstrate their unhappiness. To compound the issue, many psychologists are not fully conversant with CBT-health anxiety treatments, especially when there is existing comorbidity, and there is often a very long waiting list for intervention.

Many cases of health anxiety may be missed in medical settings, with only those patients demanding more tests or with frequent inappropriate medical readmissions attracting particular attention. A significant proportion of health-anxious patients become avoidant. Unlike some other patients, they do not seek further help, but still suffer considerably. They may have been discharged confidently from medical care, but been left debilitated by their fears, still convinced they have something seriously wrong and living a lifestyle designed to avoid any risk. In many circumstances this may lead to a miserable existence in which exercise is avoided completely, and in extreme cases patients become unable to leave the house. These patients may remain unidentified unless health professionals recognise the problem and ask the appropriate questions to elucidate it. How to identify these groups is discussed more fully in Chapter 3.

CHAPTER 2

The cognitive theory of health anxiety

The cognitive theory of emotion

The interaction between thoughts, emotions and the physical consequences of these, and subsequent behaviour are illustrated in the diagram below (Fig. 2.1). This is derived from Beck's original formulation (Beck *et al*, 1985), but of course the physical symptoms may include many that are not directly those of anxiety. Each element is interdependent on the others, often coloured by the particular context or specific environment in which symptoms arise. This model encapsulates the theory on which all cognitive therapy is based, although in the case of health anxiety it is modified for the specific problems associated with this condition. It illustrates to the patient not only how their fears are maintained, but also how work in any of the domains can produce benefits in all the others. Problems in all these areas are addressed during the course of therapy.

How health anxiety develops

Misinterpretation of bodily symptoms and sensations

The cognitive explanation for the development of health anxiety follows directly from the tendency to misinterpret bodily sensations and changes as evidence of underlying serious physical illness (Salkovskis & Warwick, 1986; Warwick & Salkovskis, 1990). The impact of these misinterpretations

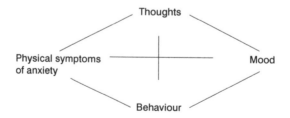

Fig. 2.1 The cognitive theory of emotion.

is dependent on the degree of threat that they carry, and how 'awful' the consequences would be for that person if they had that particular condition. The 'awfulness' does not just comprise pain and suffering, but includes wider consequences such as general disturbance of life functions, with possible inability to continue work or maintain a role within the family, especially in the longer term. Individuals with health anxiety may acknowledge that the risk to them may be tiny, but it is hugely magnified by the awfulness component, usually inflated far beyond the likelihood of illness. If the risk of developing the feared disease is much higher, for example where there is a strong family history of breast cancer, the consequent anxiety generated can be completely overwhelming.

This is further modulated by the patient's perceived ability to cope in this situation, as well as the possibility of treatment. To complicate matters further, the treatment may be perceived as almost worse than the disease, for example, where the side-effects of chemotherapy include hair loss and prolonged episodes of nausea and vomiting.

These inter-relationships can be expressed in the so-called 'Beck's equation' (Beck *et al*, 1985) (Fig. 2.2).

$$\text{Anxiety} = \frac{\text{Perceived likelihood of illness} \times \text{Perceived cost, awfulness and burden of illness}}{\text{Perceived ability to cope with illness} + \text{Perception of extent to which external factors will help}}$$

Fig. 2.2 Beck's equation.

These considerations are the same for other anxiety disorders and indeed for normal anxiety. The cognitive–behavioural approach to treating high health anxiety has the potential to address all four components of this equation (i.e. reduce likelihood and awfulness and increase coping abilities and external support), with development of specific strategies for dealing with the misconceptions in each area. This then leads to an overall reduction in anxiety (Beck *et al*, 1985).

Origins of underlying misconceptions

The tendency to develop misconceptions about health is influenced by knowledge and previous experience of disease. This includes assumptions about how diseases may present and progress. These may be coloured by perceived factors of vulnerability such as 'I've always had a weak chest' or 'There's a lot of heart disease in the family'. The first manifestation of health anxiety often tends to be in response to a trigger, such as illness or death within the family (Barsky & Klerman, 1983), at a time of stress or serious illness, or associated with a health scare in the media. At other times it may be more dramatic, with a specific health-related incident challenging previously adaptive attitudes to health. Thus, for example, take the case of an unexpected finding being demonstrated during a routine screening procedure, such as cervical cytology. Here the discovery of the abnormality, alarming enough in itself, may be made worse by the very fact that this was unexpected. More worrying to the patient is the concern that, but for the screening, the condition would have remained undetected, and this can lead to excessive monitoring of other aspects of their health.

Misconceptions are at the heart of abnormal health anxiety and are central to understanding what needs to be done in treatment. Exploring these with the patient is one of the essentials of treatment. A normal assumption about health could be, for example, a prolonged bout of significant pain that might be felt to require further investigation if it persists, whereas a maladaptive assumption might be that every minor bodily sensation constitutes the first sign of disease and requires immediate investigation. These health-anxious thoughts and the consequent anxiety generated lead to autonomic arousal (the physical accompaniments of anxiety). If the symptoms of arousal, such as sweating, dry mouth, shortness of breath and fear of the worst happening are then themselves misinterpreted as an immediate threat to health, a panic attack is the likely outcome. If, however, the symptoms are recognised as anxiety, or as is more usually the case, interpreted as early signs of the feared underlying disease, overt panic is less likely, but persistent preoccupation and worry set in, with the continued state of autonomic arousal perpetuating the sense of ill health and the conviction that there is something seriously wrong. There is, however, overlap between the two, and in later stages of health anxiety, panic attacks may coexist as the feared health outcome is perceived as drawing closer.

Everyone can experience concern about health, and may misinterpret health-related information, imagining that things may be worse than they are, but these fears tend to resolve. Even stronger worries and concerns, sometimes called 'catastrophic misinterpretations', may occur, but are usually transient. What makes these misinterpretations persist in the health-anxious patient is the way the patient reacts and responds to the perception of threat. The emphasis and precise nature of these vary from patient to patient but fall into four main areas: biases in information processing, interaction with bodily sensations, safety-seeking behaviours and the effect on mood.

Factors that maintain health anxiety

Biases in information processing

This is a more accurate description of a common fault, getting the message wrong. Those patients who develop health anxiety adopt an over-cautious approach, where, 'just to be sure', they tend to focus on health information consistent with their feared diagnosis, disregarding evidence to the contrary. This is known as 'confirmatory bias'. In addition, some patients feel they need to worry continually about their health, monitoring things closely to protect themselves from developing illness. This often takes the form of 'selective attention', when the patient automatically tunes in to bodily sensations and changes that they attribute to the feared medical condition. For example, someone with a fear of heart disease may begin to notice occasional episodes of palpitations related to exertion, forgetting that the rest of the time these are absent. Once this fear gains a hold, the patient frequently becomes hypervigilant, and starts to look out for other supporting evidence, misinterpreting other normal bodily sensations or other changes such as getting out of breath when climbing a steep staircase, confirming in their mind further evidence of the disease.

The bias in information selection can also extend to misinterpreting statements made by health professionals in the course of a consultation. For example, the doctor may say, 'There is no evidence here that suggests you have anything serious like cancer', a statement that is meant to be reassuring. However, the intensely worried patient may only hear the word 'cancer' and misinterprets what the doctor has said as 'The doctor thinks I might have cancer now!'.

Recognition of such bias and attendant maintaining behaviour is directly addressed in CBT.

Interaction with bodily sensations

Fears about health lead to an increased level of anxiety with all its associated physical symptoms. The resulting symptoms such as nausea, palpitations, shortness of breath and blurred vision are then misinterpreted as further evidence of disease. When this process occurs rapidly and the bodily sensations are interpreted catastrophically, the result will be a panic attack (Salkovskis & Clark, 1993; Salkovskis et al, 1996), but less catastrophic interpretations can still be very worrying, leading to perpetuation of symptoms. These may be identical to the symptoms generated by excitement or anger but it is their special significance that links them to the fear. There may also be selection, or specificity, in the symptoms generated, where those perceived as related to the feared disease appear to predominate. The combination of selective attention to certain bodily sensations and the perceived need to monitor health can lead to a hypersensitivity to bodily sensations and changes, and health-anxious patients tend to report some of these more accurately (Tyrer et al, 1980). For example, a patient who is anxious about having a heart attack is likely to detect symptoms of anxiety such as palpitations and a rapid pulse rate rather than other signs of anxiety and monitor these more closely. Their anxiety then increases and they continue to check their pulse rate repeatedly.

Specific strategies are developed in CBT to demonstrate the links with physiological symptoms of anxiety and to show how exploring alternative, less threatening explanations along with altering certain behaviours can lead to a reduction in these symptoms.

Safety-seeking behaviours

These can take the form of avoidance or escape behaviours intended to avert or reduce the impact of the perceived threat (Salkovskis, 1989, 1996; Salkovskis et al, 1996), but, of course, may also be a normal response to threat. So, for example, someone fearing they may develop heart disease might exercise less to avoid putting their heart under too much strain, or repeatedly attend the doctor's surgery requesting a further electrocardiogram, just in case new changes have surfaced since the last time it was performed. Patients often scour the internet, looking for reassurance there. These behaviours all tend to focus attention on health, or more accurately, on the feared disease. Sometimes patients test out their particular fear. For example, some may jog until they collapse with exhaustion to monitor whether they are developing angina. They can then interpret the exhaustion as further evidence of impaired cardiac function, thus increasing by their behaviour some of the symptoms they fear. What are called 'behavioural experiments' in psychological therapies are particularly relevant in addressing these issues.

Reassurance-seeking in all its guises can cause further problems. This can take the form of requests for repeated investigations, which can lead to the increased likelihood of an erroneous or false–positive result, potentially generating a huge increase in anxiety. It may also lead to variations in advice provided by different health professionals or by family and friends; this can further fuel the patient's concerns.

On top of this, the patient may misinterpret further tests initiated by their doctor, often performed at the patient's repeated request to 'reassure them', as evidence that their doctor also feels there is a more serious underlying problem. Paradoxically, despite much of the pressure coming from them, patients believe their doctor would only send them for a test if they also believed they were ill. They also tend to believe there is a test for every condition, and that the only way to exclude the feared disease is to have 'exactly the right test'. Health-anxious patients also tend to have an overinflated sense of responsibility with regard to their health, often irritating health professionals by producing exhaustive lists of 'symptoms' just in case one of these might be the clue to what is wrong.

Sometimes this idea has developed from a previous episode where the patient or a relative experienced a 'near miss' with their health, so they feel they have to guard against this ever happening again. For example, when a patient has experienced instant relief on resting following an episode of breathlessness brought on by fear, they may feel that by doing this they have narrowly avoided a heart attack. This perceived 'lucky escape' is likely to lead to repetition of the same behaviour in future, hence reinforcing their fear and sense of threat.

Identification of these overdeveloped notions of responsibility is part of the cognitive–behavioural approach to therapy and while tackling them, behavioural experiments can be designed to test out whether these safety-seeking behaviours are useful or unnecessary for the patient.

Effect on mood

Preoccupation with ill health often makes people feel depressed. This not only maintains, but sometimes increases, anxiety. In addition, depression is often accompanied by what are called 'automatic negative interpretations'. If you feel that you have, or are going to develop, a serious, possibly fatal illness, it is hardly surprising that you are going to feel depressed. Patients in this state of mind often consider themselves unlucky, with biased recollection of negative outcomes in the past and rumination over these. Such rumination about the consequences of the likely disease drives and helps maintain the sense of threat (Marcus *et al*, 2008).

The precise way in which these four factors work in maintaining health anxiety for a particular patient are highly specific and individualised, arising within the context of previous experience or other life stressors, and are coloured by the patient's personality. Nevertheless, there are common themes running through every patient's story and attention to all the maintaining features is crucial to understanding and treatment.

Errors in thinking

Health-anxious patients tend to think in ways which make it difficult for them to make reasonable, balanced judgements about their health. Selective attention has already been mentioned but patients also tend to catastrophise and jump to conclusions, imagining the worst possible outcome of a particular event. They may also overgeneralise, thinking that because one event has turned out badly, this will be true of all others; they discount times when things have turned out better than expected, often using phrases such as 'It's just my luck'.

In addition, these patients find it very difficult to manage risk and uncertainty. They often want 100% certainty that they are well, and if this cannot be guaranteed they assume they must be ill. They may also feel a sense of blame or guilt, always assuming things are their fault, or that they are to blame for their illness. Sometimes, they may feel that their illness is a punishment for things that they have done wrong in the past. When people then also experience accompanying bodily feelings of anxiety, it supports the notion that they are ill, and they conclude that because they feel so awful they must really be ill.

All these thinking errors are challenged directly in CBT, and this is taken forward in the next chapter.

Chapter messages

- The way we feel influences the way we think.
- Anxiety leads to physical (bodily) symptoms that can be interpreted as medical disease.
- If symptoms are misinterpreted cognitively they tend to persist as fears of disease.
- Reassurance leads to brief improvement only and repeated reassurance reinforces, not reduces, health anxiety.
- Laboratory and other investigations carried out to exclude pathology can often have the same undesirable effect as reassurance and make the symptoms of health anxiety worse.

CHAPTER 3

Style of therapy

This chapter may appear to overlap with Chapter 4, but it is included for good reason. One of the major problems when assessing people who have health anxiety is to use the right approach to address their concerns. If the wrong questions are asked, the patient will be immediately put off and there is a danger they will not engage in therapy. One of the advantages of training nurses and other professionals in introducing and giving CBT therapy for health anxiety is that they can frame it in a medical context and therefore make it much more acceptable. But this has to be accompanied by the right type of question and the probe questions discussed in this chapter are essential to doing this properly.

Identifying health anxiety, probe questions and scales

Identification of psychological disorder within a medical setting is especially challenging. People who are very obviously anxious, who constantly present to services with health worries, or alternatively consult repeatedly with innocuous symptoms and requests for further investigations, are relatively easily identified as having health anxiety. Others may be identified after a diagnosis of medically unexplained symptoms (commonly abbreviated to MUS) has been made, although the proportion of those with medically unexplained symptoms who have clinically significant health anxiety is only about 30%, as many with medically unexplained symptoms are extremely bothered by their symptoms but do not think they have a serious disease. Clinical suspicion alone, without direct questioning, will almost certainly miss many cases of health anxiety or at best identify them late, usually only after (negative) lengthy investigations. Health professionals also vary in their ability to recognise the condition and the confidence with which they feel able to diagnose it, being especially nervous in the face of what are potentially worrying symptoms. The development of screening instruments acceptable to staff and patients, and which can be administered easily, is desirable to aid recognition and diagnosis in these settings. Such screening instruments need to have high sensitivity (the proportion of positive cases correctly identified) and high specificity (the proportion of negative cases correctly identified) to allow confidence in their clinical use and application to research. The use of scales or questionnaires can be further enhanced by preliminary screening or 'probe' questions, which can be useful in excluding those who would definitely not qualify for the condition. These can be administered verbally before the scale is administered, or as a preliminary header to the questionnaire.

Probe questions

We have developed a set of these probe questions to introduce the possibility of worry without giving the impression that the problem was all in the patient's mind. It is extremely important to realise that, whatever the cause of the symptoms, what the patient is experiencing is 'real'; the patient is not making it up. You must also remember that the patient is likely to be extremely worried that they have a serious underlying condition that the doctor has failed to find, and what is more, their doctor may not seem sufficiently concerned. Sometimes the doctor–patient relationship has broken down completely, where the doctor feels the patient is wasting their time. This apparent reluctance to investigate further and find a cause for their problem can leave patients feeling isolated, helpless and very frightened.

The subject of worry is introduced gently by the doctor or health professional concerned with a series of questions, allowing plenty of time for the patient to respond and talk about their frustrations:

- 'Have you been very worried about this problem?'
- 'Do you tend to worry a lot about your health?'
- 'Have you ever been concerned that your problem might be more serious than what the doctors have found so far?'
- 'Do you feel that something might have been missed?'

If the patient answers in the affirmative to any of these questions you proceed to introduce the possibility of addressing the worry:

> 'Here in the department we are very interested in the extent to which our patients worry about their health. We know this causes a lot of distress and makes their problems more difficult to cope with.'

> 'It seems that you have been experiencing a great deal of worry about this, and we may be able to offer you some help for this, here in the department. This would be in addition to your normal medical care, which wouldn't be affected in any way.'

> 'Do you think you might be interested in receiving this extra help?'

You can then proceed to explain that one of your trained staff would see the patient for an hour to assess their concerns, and then take it forward to seeing them once a week to start with, moving on to once a fortnight, usually about 4–5 times, sometimes longer if you both feel that this would help.

The idea is to make the psychological help seem non-threatening, almost 'par for the course', and flexible. Patients who worry about their health often regard a referral to a psychologist or psychiatrist as a way of dismissing their problems as existing all in the mind. They want to see another doctor who will perform yet more tests and discover the underlying medical disorder. However, once the patient is engaged in successful therapy they will begin to see for themselves the benefits of addressing their problems in a different way.

You can introduce a scale to measure their health anxiety after the probe questions, and if they score highly, this can add weight to your proposal:

> 'I can see from this scale that you have been extremely worried over your health, and I am very keen that we should offer you some help with this.'

If your patient chooses to accept help, and they may need time to think it over, or discuss it with their family, it is important to offer them an appointment, preferably within 2 weeks. This shows the patient how seriously you are taking the problem, and should pre-empt further unnecessary medical intervention. There is one caveat to that: if the patient was still waiting for a further major medical investigation, the therapy should probably be postponed until after its completion.

Health anxiety scales

The three scales mentioned here are relatively brief, self-rated by patients, and easy to administer in a busy out-patient setting.

Health Anxiety Questionnaire (Lucock & Morley, 1996)

This scale has been devised for medical as well as psychiatric populations to tap a range of health-anxiety severity. It includes most cases of health anxiety and is suitable for use as a screening instrument. The scale is sensitive to change and is therefore of value in the assessment of psychological treatment. There is also a version of this scale for patients with chest pain (HAQ-CP), available from the author (H.T.) on request, in relation to a current research study (COgnitive behaviour therapy for Pain In the Chest, COPIC; contact: p.tyrer@imperial.ac.uk).

One criticism of the Health Anxiety Questionnaire is that it contains one question that seems to exclude the coexistence of underlying organic pathology: 'Do you ever feel that you have a serious illness?', but in practice, this is explained as a serious illness other than the one the patient has been diagnosed with.

Short Health Anxiety Inventory (Salkovskis et al, 2002)

This scale identifies most cases of health anxiety and is useful as a screening instrument; it is also sensitive to change. It measures health anxiety over the previous 6 months, an important criterion in diagnosis, but there is also a version for measuring health anxiety over the preceding week, which is useful for marking progress in treatment.

Schedule for Evaluating Persistent Symptoms (SEPS) (Tyrer *et al*, 2013)

This is a scale specifically designed to identify medically unexplained symptoms, and although this overlaps with health anxiety, it is much more inclusive. A score of 14 or more (range 0–27) suggests the patient has medically unexplained symptoms, rather than those which are only unexplained because the medical pathology has not been properly assessed.

Interview technique

The style of interviewing with these patients is designed to highlight particular aspects of their anxiety. Most of this is central to basic CBT, but it is important to recognise the particular problems that health-anxious people encounter when interacting with others, and how best to avoid these potential pitfalls during therapy. Special ways of interviewing and approaching the problem of health anxiety with these patients can prove both acceptable and illuminating. The approach is non-confrontational and collaborative, so if you are finding you are arguing a lot, you are getting it wrong.

Patients are gradually introduced to a new model that offers a quite different, and less threatening, account of their problems. This offers an alternative explanation for each of their specific disease convictions. For example, if the particular belief held is that of having cancer, the patient is asked to consider, using the evidence built up in therapy, the alternative belief that they are *worried* that they *might* have cancer. For the treatment to be effective, it is crucial that therapist and patient agree that therapeutic strategies should be aimed at reducing such worries rather than fruitless attempts to reduce risk of illness.

The discussion usually reaches the point where further information not currently available to the patient has to be sought. This is where behavioural experiments come in. These are information-gathering exercises which help the patient reach conclusions about the beliefs that they hold.

Introducing the therapy

The introduction to therapy should be relatively brief and straightforward, outlining the broad aims and how the treatment is structured. The details of the first assessment interview are provided in Chapter 4, but it is necessary to introduce the concept of the therapy first. A suitable introduction might go along these lines:

'The aim of this cognitive–behavioural therapy is to identify your concerns over your fears of illness, and by addressing these worries together, help you to cope better with the problem. The treatment sessions are usually for 1 hour, and the average length of treatment is about five sessions, although in some cases further treatment may be required. The first session tends to be an information-gathering exercise, as I need to understand about your medical history and the problems you have been experiencing in some depth, and then we can work on these concerns together over the next few weeks. This is a very straightforward, practical, down-to-earth therapy which is aimed at making you feel better, and doesn't make people worse. How does that sound?'

It is important to give plenty of opportunity for your patient to ask questions, and provide clear answers. Sometimes patients wish a relative, usually a spouse, to be present, and although this is at the discretion of the therapist, I feel that this can be acceded to, at least in the initial stage of therapy, as it helps to demystify the treatment. Also, as relatives have often witnessed the patient's worries first hand, it can help to set their minds at rest too.

Engaging the patient

It follows from the general principles described earlier (see pp. 16–17, Probe questions) that treatment of health anxiety needs to involve a shared understanding with the patient of the psychological basis of their problem. This is crucial, because at the beginning of therapy these patients believe that they are likely to have a serious or life-threatening illness. If this belief is held very strongly, the patient is unlikely to engage readily in psychologically (or psychiatrically) based treatment. It is not surprising that the health-anxious patient who believes that they have heart disease or cancer is reluctant to deal with this by psychological means. Instead, the patient seeks to solve their problem by strategies such as obtaining the best available medical advice and treatment. However, by demonstrating your understanding of the patient's fears, as well as the frustrations they have frequently experienced within the medical system, coupled with the fact that they can often, at one level, recognise that their fears are excessive, the therapist can begin to introduce to the patient that there may be an alternative way of understanding the difficulties they are experiencing.

The aim of treatment is to show patients how problems link to underlying fears, rather than to rule out physical illness. This process requires an early acknowledgement by the therapist that the symptoms experienced by the patient really exist, are not 'all in the mind' as may have been inferred by others, and that the treatment aims to provide a satisfactory explanation for these symptoms. To achieve this goal, treatment sessions should never become combative; questioning and collaboration are the key techniques. The achievement of a better explanation of symptoms is greatly simplified if the therapist remembers that patients' beliefs are invariably based on evidence that they find convincing. The good cognitive–behavioural therapist begins the process of challenging beliefs by discovering the observations that the patient believes to be evidence of illness; then, working collaboratively with the patient, they both consider whether there is any other evidence that would support alternative, less threatening beliefs.

The approach initially adopted is that helping the anxiety generated by these problems through CBT may make it easier for patients to cope with their problems. As therapy develops, the concept that anxiety itself is generating some of the problems gradually unfolds, but recognition that the anxiety is driving the symptoms is further down the line and needs to be discovered by the patient themselves, with the evidence gathered in therapy to add credence and underpin it. In cognitive therapy, you facilitate the patient to become the expert in evaluating their own thoughts and feelings.

Patients may still remain sceptical about help with their anxiety, in which case it is important that the therapist emphasises that in fact, nothing will be lost in trying this approach to their problems, and if they do not get better then the problem can be thought through again.

Guided discovery

This is a style of questioning where patients are encouraged to find the answers themselves, questioning their own beliefs and coming up with alternative answers. The goal is to help them think for themselves, finding answers that fit with their experience and make sense to them.

Consider this example:

Therapist: So when you notice this pain in your side what have you tried to do?

Patient: Well, I go and see Dr Jones to get some tests.

Therapist: Is that helpful?

Patient: Well, he needs to see me when I've got the pain so he can test me at the time and tell me what's wrong.

Therapist: And what does Dr Jones say?

Patient: He tells me that it's nothing to worry about.

Therapist: Does he do any tests?

Patient: No, he says all the tests were OK before.

Therapist: I see, so you go to Dr Jones, so that he can tell you what's wrong and do some tests, but he just tells you there is nothing wrong and doesn't repeat the tests. So how does that help you?

Patient: He tells me I'm all right and that's reassuring.

Therapist: How long does that reassurance last?

Patient: Until the pain is bad again, which is all the time at the moment. I think I might need to see someone else.

Therapist: Do you think they would handle it differently?

Patient: Probably not... I've already seen the other doctors in the surgery and Dr Smith was really abrupt – and made me feel I was wasting his time.

Therapist: So do you think going to the doctors for reassurance helps you in the long run?

Patient: No, it doesn't really, I suppose, nothing seems to help.

Therapist: So can we look together at a different way in which this pain is bothering you?

Patient: Yes, well, I need to do something; I can't go on like this...

Therapist: I agree.

This style of guided discovery (sometimes described as Socratic dialogue) is quite hard work for the patient and needs to be used judiciously; the patient should not end up feeling that they are being endlessly interrogated, but it does allow the patient to consider their own situation more broadly, instead of being continually trapped in tramlines of thinking and behaving centred around their particular belief.

It also needs to be purposeful on behalf of the therapist, directed towards the patient evaluating some particular way of thinking and behaving.

Helping patients to understand their emotions

A highly personalised approach lies at the core of treatment, for the same event can have different meanings for different people, or even for the same person on different occasions. It is the meaning that gives each event its particular emotional impact and the emotional problems arise because of the way the patient interprets reality. For example, hearing about someone famous dying of cancer on the news might not hold any special significance. However, if that person was the same gender and age as you and had died of the same feared disease, you might think that this constituted a greater risk for you. Not only that, but the fact that they were famous and despite having access to the 'best care' were unable to get life-saving help, could further undermine your confidence of surviving a serious problem.

Asking the patient to describe a recent episode when they have been particularly distressed, what they were doing at the time, their thoughts and what they perceived were the implications for them, and then asking them how this made them *feel* is crucial to understanding what is driving their fear. Some patients are not used to speaking in emotional terms, and may find it difficult to articulate their feelings. Sometimes, they may use euphemisms such as 'Well, it just doesn't make sense to me' or 'I'm fed up with it all', or just make frank statements such as 'I don't know how it makes me feel'. Then sensitive questioning along the lines of 'When you say the doctor doesn't seem bothered, do you feel on your own? Does that make you feel frightened?' may provide a breakthrough.

Basic structure of a CBT session

The content of therapy will vary from session to session and depend on the particular patient. An outline of the initial therapy sessions is given in Chapter 4, but some general rules are that each session should have a loose structure, last about 1 hour, including 50 minutes therapy, with time at the end to make any additional notes and to fix the next appointment.

1 *Introduction.* Here, a brief outline of what will be covered in the session is put forward (this does not have to be set in stone, but helps keep things on track and can be amended).

2 *Ask the patient whether there is anything they would like to bring up during the session,* or any issues or clarification arising out of the previous session. If there is a burning issue, perhaps a new and highly relevant problem that has arisen during the previous week, this may need to

take precedence. Some other angles the patient may want to bring up can be included, or postponed until a later appointment, but they must be carefully noted and not forgotten.

3 *If homework was set in the preceding session,* this should be asked about and discussed as an early item on the agenda (this is discussed in more detail in Chapter 6).

4 *A summary of the work that has taken place in the session should take place at the end,* cementing what has been covered and giving the patient time to raise anything they are not clear about.

5 *Finally, there should be clarification of any homework set,* which should include listening again to the session if it has been recorded for the patient. Homework setting is discussed in more detail in Chapter 6.

6 *Date, venue and time of next appointment.* At the start of therapy, appointments are usually weekly, but as therapy progresses they can be arranged at longer intervals, with some spaced out booster sessions at the end if necessary. Patients need time to make changes and see the long-term benefit, and they may experience setbacks which can be addressed while they are still in therapy.

Sometimes, patients may need to be seen at home for a variety of reasons. If this is the case, a risk assessment should be undertaken with the supervisor, and the therapist should always inform a colleague of the time and location of the appointment and check back in with them on completion.

Every effort should be made to encourage patients to keep appointments. If a patient cancels repeatedly or fails to attend, contact them by whichever means you have arranged inviting them to re-attend. Engaging in a psycho-logical therapy can be a very big step for some patients and showing that you take it seriously and are committed to helping them is very important.

Sometimes sessions are best arranged around important events, such as immediately before an important medical review, and can help the patient prepare for this. You may also be required to act as an advocate for your patient with other agencies, for example GPs, Social Services and employment review bodies.

Chapter messages

- Health anxiety cannot be identified by clinical suspicion alone and needs probe questions to bring it to the surface.
- The assessor must never give the impression that the symptoms of health anxiety are not 'real'; they are as real as any other symptoms and cause great distress.
- Ask questions to find out how the patient understands their symptoms and experiences, and allow adequate time to express these in full.
- Pick on examples of recent episodes of anxiety early in the interview so that real, not hypothetical, problems are identified and addressed.

CHAPTER 4

The initial assessment

Please note: This may be done over two sessions if needed, but it is best to complete it in one.

Introducing the patient to the therapy

Patients with health anxiety are usually sceptical about the value of psychological intervention. They may also have a diagnosed medical condition independent of their health anxiety, so you must make it clear that you are acknowledging this, even though their anxiety may be excessive. At the initial consultation they should be warmly welcomed and made comfortable. You then make a brief introduction about the reason they have been referred to you and the nature of CBT.

For example, you might begin the interview with:

'Your doctor has asked me to see you about some of the worries you have had over your health. The extent to which you worry over your health can contribute to your problems and make them more difficult to cope with. Cognitive–behavioural therapy, or CBT as it is also known [you can use the CBT abbreviation quite early on in the interview as everyone now tends to know this], helps you explore some of these fears and worries. This can help you come to terms with, and in some cases, solve some of your difficulties.'

It might be appropriate at this stage to ask whether the doctor explained the reason for the referral and also to ask whether the patient has any questions at this point. It should be stressed that the CBT treatment is an additional intervention only and will not interfere with their normal medical care. An outline of the likely number of sessions could be made at this stage.

Helping the patient feel understood

Taking a history

The assessment interview continues by emphasising the physiological concomitants of the problem and the patient's beliefs about their physical state.

Continue the interview by saying:

'I'd like to begin by finding out what's been happening recently about your health.'

Patients have often come prepared to say various things they feel you may need to know, and it is important to let them explain these. This need not take long, but often these patients have become accustomed to being cut short, and they often feel that unless the doctor has listened to every tiny aspect of their problem they will miss a vital clue to the correct diagnosis. So, if you do need to curtail what your patient is saying, explain that the information they are telling you is really important, but that you will need to take this down properly later, and it often helps to let the patient see that you are making a note to do that. You can also ask the patient to make a complete list of their problems which they can bring to the next visit.

The next stage is to take a relatively brief medical history. You should have already looked through their medical records, or have some information regarding their medical problems. This will comprise an account of when their (medical) problems first started, what appointments and investigations they have had and what the doctor has given in the way of explanation, and how they have interpreted this. You also need to ask how long they have been worrying about their health. This may be lifelong or related to more recent events. You then summarise this information briefly for the patient to make sure it is correct before proceeding.

It is very important during this history-taking to realise how distressing the recent problems may have been for the patient and throughout this process, be able to reflect on subjects or events that are particularly sensitive, sometimes noting what the patient says verbatim. For example, 'Doctor X told me when I asked about the ECG changes that they were of the sort that could kill you'. You respond by acknowledging that this must have been extremely frightening and 'flag this up' by noting it down.

Within medical settings it is also common to find that many mixed messages have been given. The patient may have seen different doctors, not just as a result of emergency admissions, but also within out-patient settings. They may not see the same member of the clinical team at follow-up, or may see a locum. Training doctors also rotate fairly frequently through different jobs. Sometimes medical notes are missing or the results of investigations are not available; this may be especially true where a patient has been referred to another hospital for surgery, for example. All these things matter enormously to patients, who may have been waiting anxiously for their next appointment, which may have already been rearranged more than once. They will have been going over and over in their mind about what was said at the last appointment, or what they perceived was said, as they may also have misunderstood things, or remembered things incorrectly.

Health-anxious patients particularly tend to home in on emotive words such as 'growth' or 'tumour', so if the consultant were to say, 'It's very unlikely this is a growth in your lung, but we need to do a few baseline investigations', the patient may interpret that as, 'He thinks there is a growth there! Why is he only doing baseline investigations? When are the other tests going to be done?'. If this patient then finds at their follow-up appointment that not only are they seeing a different, more junior-looking doctor, but that in addition some of the test results are missing, they are likely to be very upset and even more anxious, particularly if the doctor does not seem too concerned.

Sometimes health-anxious patients also imagine that test results have not come back because there was something seriously wrong with them and the pathologist or radiographer needs to look at them more closely. Tests can also be mislaid or inconclusive and need repeating, and, of course, this becomes another major source of concern. In addition, some health-anxious patients fail to believe negative results, fearing that the result may have been muddled up with that of someone else in some way.

Sometimes, a patient may have had a working diagnosis with a condition such as angina, and been prescribed a raft of different medications, but subsequently the results of a treadmill test and other investigations suggest all is clear. Far from being reassured, the patient may feel angry at what they perceive as a misdiagnosis and failure of medical care. They may feel puzzled over the prescription of medication, particularly as the tablets might now be stopped, leaving the patient angry that they had not needed them in the first place. Alternatively, the medication may be continued as prophylaxis against future heart disease without clear explanation, leaving the patient wondering why they still need to be taking them.

Doctors may have had no idea that a patient has been left confused, and are often working under considerable time pressure in very busy clinics. It is also true that patients frequently do not question things at the time, sometimes because they feel unable to, but often because it is only when they get home that they struggle to make sense of things.

It is very important to help the patient feel acknowledged and understood, and chart these problems, empathising with them ('That must have been very worrying for you...') and asking the patient how they felt at the time, validating their feelings and concerns. In addition, for some of these patients, the relationship with their doctor has been severely tested or has broken down because of their repeated demands for reassurance. Helping the patient to feel understood and be able to express what they feel is at the heart of CBT for health anxiety.

Evaluation of any symptoms and their interpretation by the patient

The next stage of the interview is to list the patient's symptoms, preferably using the following format:

a   listing all their symptoms on the left-hand side of a piece of paper;
b   writing down what each symptom means for the patient on the right-hand side;

c   deciding which symptoms are the most important to the patient (see below).

Some patients may have very little in the way of symptoms and their problems are essentially caused by the fear of symptoms developing now or at some time in the future. Others will have a multitude of symptoms or complaints that bother them.

It is crucial that patients feel that all their symptoms have been considered, as often they have not been allowed to describe them in any depth in the past. This may have been because of essentials-only history-taking, time pressures, or when the patient has been a frequent attender; the interviewer may feel that they have said it all before. This is usually accompanied by the suspicion that the doctor has already made up their mind that there is nothing significantly wrong or new. Although succinct history-taking works for most patients, in those who are health anxious it may increase their fear that something significant may have been missed.

If there seems to be an endless list of symptoms, write down all those that are considered to be of reasonable importance and ask the patient to provide a list of the others for the next appointment. However, if the patient has already brought a list of the symptoms to the meeting, it is important that this is acknowledged and the patient understands that they have all been noted. If at any time the patient seems to be providing information too quickly, it is quite acceptable to ask them to pause – 'Could I ask you to stop there for a moment as it is quite important that I get this down properly?' – so that due weight is given to every complaint. This reinforces the notion that the patient is being taken seriously.

For each symptom, it is necessary to elicit what exactly this means for the patient. This may require some teasing out of the details, as in the past these symptoms may have been ridiculed or airily dismissed. In some cases, the patient may find it difficult to use certain words, such as 'cancer'. It is also possible that the patient has never actually considered the specific nature of the symptom; the meaning then may come over in abstract form. For example, a patient may describe stomach pain on the left-hand side of the body in the following terms:

Therapist: When you have this pain, what do you think it might mean?
Patient: I don't know really.
Therapist: What do you think might be causing it?
Patient: Well, the doctor says it's nothing serious but I keep getting it.
Therapist: Do *you* feel it might be something serious?
Patient: It seems very likely, doesn't it?
Therapist: So do you think it might be an infection or a growth like cancer, or another serious medical condition?
Patient: Yes, I think it might be something like that.
Therapist: Can you be more specific and let me know exactly what you fear?
[There is a long pause]
Patient: I am really frightened that it's bowel cancer.

Sometimes these discussions can create distress and the patient may begin to cry. This is important, as it shows you have reached a core fear that will need to be addressed in therapy. It may be the first time the patient has ever expressed this fear directly and it should be received with sympathy and understanding. So in response to the patient saying that they have a fear of cancer, say something along the lines of: 'When you have this pain you think it might be cancer? This must be really frightening for you.'

Patients who are very anxious are often preoccupied with thoughts about what will eventually happen to them, although such thoughts can be very difficult to elicit. This difficulty is especially marked when patients are actively trying not to dwell on their fears. For example, a patient whose key complaint is headache may say it is there all the time but they try not to think of it. When asked whether they can remember anything that makes the problem worse or better, or whether they have noticed any patterns according to the day of the week, time of the month or time of the year, they may be able to remember how they interpreted the pain at those times. Did their opinion of the cause of the pain vary, and what went through their mind when the pain was particularly bad? Consider an example of a patient's symptoms and their interpretation in Table 4.1.

The therapist should enquire about visual images related to the problem. For example, a patient who complained of shortness of breath was able to identify a visual image of choking for breath as they were dying; this image was associated with an increase in both anxiety and perceived breathlessness. Assessment of the perceived cost of illness usually involves the therapist probing the patient's beliefs about what would happen if they did develop the disease that they feared. For example, the therapist might say:

'You are obviously very afraid of cancer. To find out more about this fear, can you remember the last time you felt it was very likely that you did indeed have cancer? At that particular time, when you were worrying about cancer, how did you see it developing? What seemed to be especially awful about having cancer? What would it be like for you and for the people you love?'

Table 4.1 Symptoms and their meaning attributed by patient (example)

Symptom	Meaning
Cough	'Severe lung disease or possibly cancer. I've left it too long, so they won't be able to treat it'
Feeling short of breath	'My lungs are permanently damaged now'
Backache	'It could be arthritis or secondary cancer in the spine, I might even be riddled with cancer!'
Abdominal pain	'An ulcer, or liver failure, or a growth, but they won't be able to treat this because my lungs won't stand the anaesthetic. My uncle died when he had an operation and that was just for a hernia!'

Further probes obviously depend on the specific answers given by the patient. The perceived consequences of illness are particularly upsetting for patients, who are often reluctant to describe their fears in great detail. Throughout the assessment and treatment, empathy and understanding are crucial, particularly at this stage. Frequent summarising of both the information and its emotional impact is helpful in encouraging patients to focus on this material, and also has the effect of normalising the reactions and reinforcing the formulation that is being developed. For example, the therapist might summarise by saying:

> 'So it's really not surprising that you are so upset about these lumps under your arms. Not only do you think that they mean you have cancer, but you also believe that cancer will kill you slowly and painfully, that you will lose your dignity, and that your family will suffer terribly both before and after your eventual death. You believe that your young daughter's life will be totally destroyed. These are really terrifying ideas. How do you think someone else who had these beliefs would react? Do you think that the person might behave in the same way as you?'

It is also important to realise that patients often have multiple fears and this exercise gives an overall picture of the extent of what is troubling them. This is expanded as therapy progresses.

You now want to ask them what their worst symptom/fear is and for them to try to remember a recent episode when this was particularly distressing. At this point, summarise with the patient what you have understood from their list of symptoms and meanings, adding any other comments that the patient may make at this point that are felt to be useful. This exercise of taking together all the patient's experiences and fears about their health helps the patient, probably for the first time, to feel understood. You are then ready to move to the formulation.

Moving to a formulation

The formulation is the keystone to understanding and beginning therapy. It requires time and patience to construct, and is intended to build a full picture of how symptoms, fears and beliefs, and maintaining factors link together. It usually takes at least 30 minutes, and is either completed in the second half of the first session, or, if the history-taking has been protracted, in the subsequent meeting.

The formulation is built up as a flow chart together with the patient, so it is helpful if you can position yourself so the patient can clearly observe you as you construct it. In the diagram (Fig. 4.1, p. 30), boxes are included to suggest the steps and concepts involved. The actual details, however, are completely specific and personal to the patient, and an example is given with a patient I shall call Louise.

The first step is to take the patient back to a recent, particularly distressing time when they were worrying about their health. It is important to be as specific as possible about the date, the day of the week and the time of day, and what they were doing immediately before the fear set in, who was present and so on. Getting the patient to relive this episode as closely as possible enables you to elicit the full meaning that the event had for them and the fears that it generated.

During the process of developing the formulation you will often be eliciting very personal, distressing meanings and images from your patient, and they are very likely to get upset. It is crucial that you attend to these emotions, noting down – gently – exactly what is going through the patient's mind and exploring what is at the core of the fear, rather than reassuring them and moving on.

An example of this might be a patient breaking down at the thought of dying and not seeing her daughter grow up. You might gently probe further, asking:

> 'This is clearly very distressing for you, thinking you won't be there when your child grows up. That's a horrible thought. What else might that mean for you?'

The response might be that her spouse might remarry and her place as a mother would be taken by someone else, or perhaps she recalls when her mother died prematurely, or that she would never see her grandchildren, and would not be remembered. Sometimes this may take you away temporarily from the formulation, but it is important to encourage the patient to develop the thoughts they were experiencing, and much of what they tell you will be built into it. However, it is equally important to draw them back to the particular episode, noting down with them any issues you may need to come back to later.

Sometimes the patient has difficulty recalling a particular event. If this is the case, it may be necessary to concentrate on their day-to-day worries and look for an opportunity to concentrate attention on a particular time or event (Fig. 4.1).

Using Beck's equation

The formulation should provide crucial information about what is driving the fear, and the various elements that have been elicited can be built into the Beck equation (Beck et al, 1985), validating and clarifying the patient's concerns (see Fig. 2.2, p. 9).

It sometimes happens that the patient accepts that certain conditions are rare, but for them the consequences of that event occurring would be so dreadful (the concept of 'perceived awfulness' from Beck's equation) that this outweighs the low level of perceived likelihood of illness. The denominators of the equation could also be reduced; the person may feel quite unable to cope with the symptoms, they might experience overwhelming pressure for safety-seeking behaviours such as seeking reassurance. The tests may be perceived as threatening or intolerable and so on. All this can be worked back into the formulation to explain why the patient's fear persists.

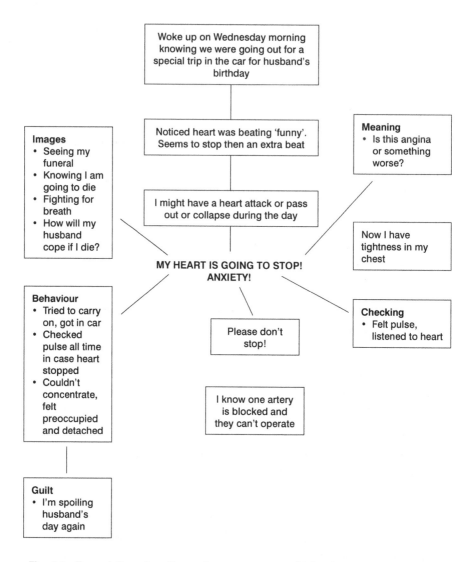

Fig. 4.1 Formulation of an illustrative recent event with Louise.

For some important fears, the equation is so heavily weighted towards awfulness that the low likelihood of a particular illness occuring is almost ignored. 'If it did occur,' the patient thinks, 'it would be so dreadful that I must do everything in my power to prevent it from happening'. Putting the fear into this sort of context can help greatly in evaluating related symptoms. You can build on this further by emphasising the low likelihood of the disease occurring, boosting the top part of the equation by using the pie chart or pyramid methods described in Chapter 5, and the effects of checking, techniques with which they may now be familiar or which you can introduce. You can also help to diminish the awfulness of the fear by discussing better coping strategies, for example, asking the patient whether they can remember a time when they had to cope with a very difficult situation in the past. What did they do and how did they manage then? You can also diminish the importance of a symptom or feared illness by discussing what treatments are available. Patients often feel that treatments are less effective than they actually are, and have given preferential attention to scare stories in the media. They therefore tend to underestimate the value of medical intervention. This can be discussed and examples drawn out and used to reduce the importance of the symptom. You may be able to identify examples of successful medical help from the patient's own experience or of other people they know. Their tendency to pay selective attention to negative outcomes can therefore be reduced.

The equation is usefully introduced fairly early on, with an explanation that all elements of it will be addressed in therapy. You can personalise it, then refer back to it, challenging the beliefs in each component as therapy helps build up evidence of less threatening conclusions.

In our example, Louise was aware that she had a degree of ischaemic heart disease, so the likelihood of having further problems was already magnified. The perceived awfulness was the thought of dying, and for her that meant knowing the *exact* moment at which she would die, gasping for breath. This was a vivid image and truly horrific for her; coupled with that was the thought of her husband struggling to cope without her, his life ruined. So when she experienced the palpitations (subsequently demonstrated by diary techniques to be almost exclusively generated by anxiety) she was overwhelmed with fear that she was about to die from a heart attack. This was compounded by the feelings that she could not cope with her fear and would never cope with not being able to breathe properly. Her only way of attempting to manage the problem would be to 'listen' to her heart under all circumstances, and continually monitor her pulse, which of course would be completely counterproductive, focusing attention on her problem all the time. In addition, Louise felt external factors, such as treatment, might not be available to her, and this was in fact true with regard to some potential surgical interventions such as bypassing the blocked coronary artery, as she had a blood-clotting disorder that rendered such a procedure too dangerous.

Seeing the equation 'filled in' for her situation made it quite clear, for the first time really, how her fear was generated and maintained; it all made sense. It also made sense that we needed to address all aspects of the equation in therapy. When this was gradually achieved, we were able to re-write the text, with her putting lines through the original conclusions and substituting more rational – less threatening – beliefs in their place. Broadly, this comprised building evidence that she did not have very severe heart disease, and when she had had her angiogram the cardiologist had been unconcerned about her palpitations (see Chapter 10 for managing health anxiety in cardiology clinics). This, along with the diary, provided evidence that the two were unrelated. We also explored the fact that no one knew the exact moment they were going to die, and if she were killed in a car accident the next day, she could think of all the ways in which her husband would in fact be able to cope, using examples of when he had coped with difficult situations before, as well as all the support other family and friends would supply, and their relatively secure financial position.

Regarding the treatment or 'rescue factors', Louise concluded that she was in fact now in a better place, as she was on prophylactic medication for heart disease and hyperlipidaemia and had had other more serious problems excluded by investigations. She realised that there was no need to monitor her health herself as she was being followed up appropriately for her problem within a recognised programme of care. This released her from problematic, constant checking, which we had demonstrated only served to increase her anxiety. Of course, both these conclusions also helped her realise that this too meant she was at reduced likelihood of a serious cardiac event.

Louise was able to work on all four aspects of the equation, and as a consequence realised her position was much less threatening. This process helped to reduce her anxiety, and by getting the situation in proportion she gradually felt safer and was able to get back to a normal life.

Recording and summarising

A lot of work is carried out within each session, both in gaining understanding and in generating new ideas. It is crucially important to write these down with the patient. You are effectively helping them to keep important notes about their beliefs and new understandings to which they will need to refer. It is also incredibly valuable to flag up particular concerns, insights or valuable conclusions that your patient comes to. These can be huge markers of realisation and progress, and need to be validated on the page. You will almost certainly find it useful to refer back to these comments in the future and if not recorded, valuable material can be lost.

In addition, it can be extremely valuable to make audio recordings of the sessions, both for the patient and therapist to listen to again; they are also helpful for evaluation of therapy and supervision. When patients are able to listen again to a therapy session, it serves to jog their memory and maximise the therapeutic input, cementing the progress they have made. It can also be revelatory for the patient to hear themselves voicing their fears; some patients comment that they cannot believe that they sounded so negative, and others have said that they had not realised how ridiculous some of their beliefs were until they heard them articulated back. For the occasional patient, they have never spoken their thoughts out loud before and this can help them confront their fears. For the therapist, when listening again, new things can strike you which need addressing; there may have been an important piece of information which you missed or a comment made which reveals new insight on the problem. It can also highlight when the patient has not quite followed what you have said, or how you might have explained something more clearly. It can help you to become more focused and efficient in your style.

Towards the end of the session leave sufficient time to go over the work you have done, summarising the main points of the discussion. It is important to do this with reference to the notes you have made, clarifying any confusing points. You will be asking the patient to look through their copy of the work they have done as part of their homework. If you are unsure how much the patient has understood at any stage, ask them to summarise what you have just said. For example, you could gently ask questions such as: 'What did you feel were the main things that we covered today? Shall we go through these notes together? Can you follow what I've put down here? Does this make sense to you?'.

Homework-setting

Patients have often suffered with their fears for a considerable time and they have often become all-encompassing, entrenched and difficult to shift. One hour of therapy a week, no matter how well delivered, is unlikely to be sufficient if nothing is put in place between sessions to supplement the work done. Going over the work completed in the last therapy session, by reading through the notes you made together and listening to any recording you have made, is mandatory and constitutes the bare minimum. Following the initial therapy sessions, additional reading material may be required in the form of handouts explaining the nature of health anxiety and how it is maintained, but it may well include the patient attempting another formulation for another episode of fear, either completed at the time, or, if they are too distressed to do it then, to be completed later in the evening or the next day. They may also think of other aspects they could add to the formulation you have already done. Patients should be encouraged to do this, writing things in, as this serves to give them ownership of their work.

Sometimes, patients who find it particularly difficult to get in touch with their emotions or to remember how they felt at a particular time, can be advised to keep a diary of events, their thoughts at the time and how it made them feel over the succeeding week, and to bring it along to the next session. To encourage them to do this, it is important to provide them with a table to fill in, helping them to start it off with a few examples, such as:

> *Therapist:* Let's think about the situation of coming here today, when you were on the way here, what was going through your mind?
>
> *Patient:* Well, I didn't know what to expect, in fact I nearly rang and cancelled.
>
> *Therapist:* That's understandable. So how were you feeling about it inside?
>
> *Patient:* Nervous, apprehensive really and a little bit sick.

Then you help them to start filling in a table in the format of Table 4.2, exploring the relationship between events and the thoughts and feelings that surround them.

Table 4.2 Table to link events to thoughts and feelings

Situation	Thoughts	Feelings
On the way to first therapy session	I didn't know what to expect	Felt nervous, apprehensive, a bit sick
Talking to boss at work about an encountered problem	He'll think I'm stupid and inadequate	Worried and miserable
...	...	...

Whatever homework you have set, it is absolutely crucial to ask about it at the following visit, otherwise it is completely devalued and the patient is unlikely to complete any in the future.

Chapter 6 covers homework setting in more detail.

Chapter messages

- Always allow the patient full opportunity to describe their symptoms in detail, and if you are in a hurry, make sure that adequate time is made available later.
- Find out what each symptom means for the patient.
- Identify the worst symptom wherever possible.
- Use the last time the worst symptom occurred to start making a formulation.
- Use the Beck equation liberally; do not feel inhibited by bringing it up whenever you feel like doing so to put the interpretation of a symptom into proportion.

CHAPTER 5

Specific techniques

The essence of CBT is to encourage patients to identify their dysfunctional thoughts, beliefs and unhelpful behaviours, enable them to generate less threatening alternatives and then test them out. With health anxiety there is a tendency to overestimate the possibility of ill health, accompanied by the need to monitor health excessively in all the various forms that may take. The next sessions of treatment should include guidance on specific techniques to address these problems, particularly exploring how health anxiety is generated and fuelled, encouraging ways to achieve a more normal perspective on health and to put in place ways of maintaining this.

Techniques that help to alter distorted perceptions

Pie charts

The pie chart technique is helpful in two ways. First, it helps to generate non-serious, less threatening, alternative explanations for the patient's particular complaint, and it also helps put that complaint in perspective by working out the frequency of non-serious conditions.

The pie chart can be introduced by saying:

> 'Let's make a pie chart of all possible causes of the particular symptom/ sensation that is troubling you.'

Thus, for example, if a patient's main cause for concern is an intermittent dry throat/cough, and they conclude that they have untreatable lung cancer, you jointly make a list of all the causes of a dry cough (remember, in this exercise we try to get the patient, not the therapist, to make most of the suggestions), which will of course include lung cancer, but should also include many less serious or non-serious causes; some basic medical knowledge can be helpful here. The severe, potentially life-threatening causes are best incorporated under one heading, avoiding the generation of a long list of severe illnesses. An example of such a list is given in Box 5.1. The idea is to generate so many innocuous causes in addition to the serious ones that it becomes apparent that the most serious outcome is the least likely.

Box 5.1   Serious and innocuous causes of dry cough – examples

- Life-threatening conditions such as lung cancer and AIDS
- Tuberculosis
- Asthma/allergies
- Cough and cold
- Smoking (ask whether the patient smokes – surprisingly many health-anxious patients do)
- Catarrh
- Irritants in the air/clearing the throat
- Alcohol (there is usually a place for this on every list!)
- Clearing your throat (e.g. when everyone coughs between pieces in a concert)
- Throat infection
- Laryngitis
- Exercise (e.g. running)

The pie chart is then filled up by asking, of all the people in a certain locality (usually the patient's local town) who have a cough, what proportion would be affected by the particular causes itemised on the list. This can be done in two ways, either starting with the most innocuous causes first, or, if the most serious causes are at the top of the list, starting at the bottom. With the latter method you can seem to avoid bias in the patient's eyes. The first method can be introduced as: 'Let's look at the common things first'. This helps flag up the fact that some conditions are more common than others and will make sense to the patient. So the therapist might ask: 'How many people might cough from time to time to clear their throat?'. The answer might come back that as this was a very common phenomenon it might be 40%; this proportion of the pie chart is then filled in. There should be a similarly large percentage for coughs and colds, catarrh, and laryngitis and other relatively minor conditions, and so the pie chart becomes rapidly filled up, leaving little or no space for the more serious causes, let alone the life-threatening alternatives. These should come out around 1% or less (an example of a pie chart is given in Fig. 5.1).

The 'life-threatening' group of causes can then be further broken down into those conditions that are serious but treatable, those that are difficult to treat, those that are untreatable and of the last, what are the conditions that are uniformly fatal. The last group is very small indeed, thereby indicating to the patient that the likelihood of a cough being due to lung cancer is very small.

This technique helps the patient build up alternative explanations for worrying symptoms. Previously, they will usually have linked a symptom immediately to the most feared outcome and been unable to think of any other explanation. This new approach helps them acquire a sense of proportion, and importantly, because it has been done in a collaborative

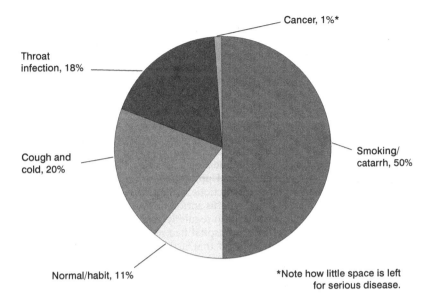

Fig. 5.1 Pie chart for cough.

manner with the patient thinking about and generating innocuous symptoms for themselves, as well as working out how very common they are, the final pie chart represents the patient's own conclusions. This exercise is often a complete revelation to the patient, who previously has never been able to consider any other alternative diagnosis for their particular symptom, and of course it can be repeated for other symptoms or sensations they experience.

Patients should be encouraged to study the pie chart (leave a copy with them) as part of their homework, and to refer back to it when they experience that particular symptom again. However, as this is a collaborative exercise (certainly initially), it could prove impossible or even backfire if the patient were to attempt it on their own, as they may be unable to think up sufficient innocuous examples for a new symptom. In time they should develop this skill, after practising with other examples of common symptoms and when they have progressed in therapy.

Pie charts can also be useful in other ways. Patients with persistent health anxiety tend to feel a heightened sense of responsibility regarding their health, as an attempt to guard against developing a disease they fear. Consequently, they have to be constantly on the lookout for bodily symptoms and signs, or may feel the need to closely monitor an existing illness, which usually manifests itself by excessive checking and reassurance-seeking. In these cases, a pie chart apportioning responsibility can be helpful, where a list of the agencies involved in monitoring can be fitted into the pie.

Let us take Case example 5.1.

Case example 5.1: A man with glaucoma

A 60-year-old man with high health anxiety had had a malignant tumour behind his eyeball treated with a radioactive implant. A complication of this was that he had developed a degree of glaucoma (a potentially severe problem of raised pressure within the eyeball), and was terrified he might lose the sight in that eye or that the disease might spread to the other eye. In an effort to monitor this he would check his ability to read car number plates from a distance many times a day, first with one eye, then the other. This led to considerable anxiety, especially as the cars could be at varying distances and so any discrepancy immediately led to further checking. When asked about the hospital care, he said it was excellent and he agreed that they kept regular checks on him in line with recommended guidelines. He also agreed that his optician, who had originally picked up that there was a problem, saw him regularly. When asked what instructions he had been given by the hospital, he explained that he had had to put his antibiotic eye drops in religiously after the surgery, and take his medication regularly, and attend his appointments. When asked, he agreed that the hospital had never asked him to personally monitor his vision. He also agreed that if there was a deterioration in his vision he would pick it up anyway as he had before.

In this case, the pie chart was filled up with the agencies most responsible for his care being inserted first: 95% was apportioned to the consultant and his team in the ophthalmology department, and the rest was spread between the optician and the GP. In this way, he could see that checking the car number plates was completely superfluous to his medical requirements, and he was able to cease this activity with confidence; this was followed by an immediate reduction in the attendant anxiety.

Pie charts can also be used in this way for the overdeveloped sense of personal responsibility for things going wrong, which is one of the underlying features of obsessive–compulsive disorder (OCD).

For patients with chronic pain (see Chapter 16), a pie chart can be constructed of all the ways in which their life is affected by the pain, with the proportions decided by the patient. The patient can then consider each portion and think which of them they may be able to do something about. In this way the problem can be broken down and the patient can begin to exercise some measure of control.

Pyramids

Patients with high health anxiety tend to overestimate the seriousness of symptoms. The pyramid technique, similar to the pie chart, helps to challenge these beliefs and quantify such risks more appropriately. It is particularly useful for those patients who experience a lot of bodily sensations or changes that are immediately interpreted as catastrophic, serving to illustrate how very rarely a common complaint with which a patient presents to their GP turns out to be anything serious. It achieves this by emphasising the gradual steps in medical care, from first presenting with a problem to that problem possibly being confirmed as evidence of a terminal, untreatable disease. The base of the pyramid represents all patients with that particular symptom, with each subsequent rising level representing more progressively negative outcomes. Eventually, the apex is reached, representing the very tiny proportion of those patients initially presenting who end up with a life-threatening, untreatable disease. The patient is asked to estimate the proportion of patients who rise to each level, demonstrating to themselves that most symptoms or bodily sensations have non-threatening outcomes. See Case example 5.2.

Case example 5.2: A troublesome cough

Jack, aged 21, had a fear that he had or was going to develop throat cancer. Despite this, he continued to smoke cannabis, which contained some tobacco, and cigarettes, as he felt there was no point stopping because it was 'too late'. He had developed high health anxiety following the death of his father from heart disease 2 years previously, experiencing a series of different health concerns and very frequent visits to his GP and various consultants. He had had a lingering cough for 6 weeks following an upper respiratory tract infection over the Christmas period, and despite repeated reassurance from his GP, who had seen many similar cases over the winter, he was anxious to be referred to an ear, nose and throat (ENT) specialist for a second opinion. He took every opportunity to look in the mirror for any lumps or distortion to his neck, and continually felt for lumps. The GP had examined his neck and throat on many occasions, finding no abnormality.

The GP asked Jack to consider how many people might have visited their doctor with a troublesome cough over the winter period (a considerable number). He was then asked of the last 100 who had attended, represented within a bar drawn across the bottom of a page, how many would the GP need to see again because they were still unwell. Jack estimated about 20% (a figure the GP considered inflated, but the importance of the exercise was to let his patient reach his own conclusions). The GP then drew a bar 20% of the width of the original above it. He then asked his patient to consider what percentage of this 20% who had had to return might require further investigations rather than reassurance or medication. It was discussed that these further investigations might be blood tests, a swab or a chest X-ray, and Jack estimated this to be about 5%, and an appropriately sized bar was drawn above the other two. As illustrated in the diagram from this case (Fig. 5.2), he was asked to consider how many of those tests would come back abnormal, how many of those would require referral, how many of those patients would have significant disease, and of those, what percentage would be serious and, finally, untreatable. The conclusion is that a minute percentage of the original patients with the troublesome cough had anything potentially serious, let alone untreatable.

Jack found this quite revealing, but said he still felt that he might be the one at the top of the pyramid, so he was asked to do a similar exercise, as homework, for all the other symptoms that had worried him over the 2 years. This included thinking he had had a lump in his testicle which was cancer, a rash on his arm, which he had also thought was due to malignancy, headaches from time to time, and bouts of abdominal pain. When the conclusions were the same in each case, he was able to accept that most conditions that GPs see tend to settle on their own with minimal intervention, and on reflection, this was possibly true for him too. It was opening up a less threatening explanation for his cough. It then became apparent that part of his coughing was deliberate in order to check what it sounded like, and once he resisted that, armed by his increased confidence that it might not be so serious, it quickly disappeared.

He concluded he no longer needed to see a specialist as it would be a waste of time. He also decided (successfully) to stop smoking cigarettes and dramatically reduced his cannabis use.

Identifying patterns of mood and behaviour: keeping a diary

A lot of patients, when asked about their fears and anxiety say that they are worried all the time, and they cannot readily or reliably identify times when it is worst, or it can be difficult to identify anything other than the most obvious triggers. When worry is accompanied by alarming symptoms, health-anxious patients tend to assume that the symptoms are the cause of the worry, and to some extent this is true, for when the symptoms appear they become a cause for concern. However, it is often the case that the anxiety has triggered the physical problem, as it was the anxiety that came first. This is an important distinction to make, for if it is identified that the worrying symptoms are generated by anxiety, it builds the case that it is fear of underlying disease that is the problem, rather than an actual disease, or relapse of a former disease. This allows for a less threatening interpretation of the particular symptom or sensation.

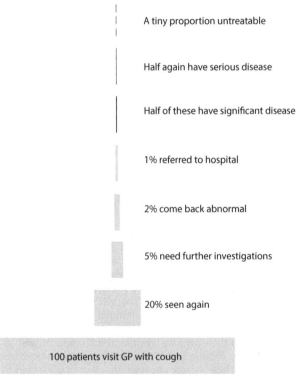

A tiny proportion untreatable

Half again have serious disease

Half of these have significant disease

1% referred to hospital

2% come back abnormal

5% need further investigations

20% seen again

100 patients visit GP with cough

Fig. 5.2 The pyramid for causes of cough.

Keeping a diary of events, symptoms and anxiety levels is a means of identifying this. See Case example 5.3.

Case example 5.3: Non-cardiac chest pain

John was a middle-aged man who had been promoted at work, despite some recent redundancies at the factory. He was finding his new role as a manager uncomfortable on several counts: he had much more paperwork, some of which he did not properly understand, he now had to discipline his old mates on the shop floor (and as a consequence, took sandwiches for lunch which he ate alone in his office, rather than joining his colleagues in the canteen like he used to) and in addition, he had to prepare forecasts and reports for the senior management team and present them at the 'team meeting' on Monday and Thursday mornings.

Two years previously, his elderly father had died of a heart attack. Shortly afterwards John was admitted twice with episodes of chest pain. All investigations at the time were negative, apart from the recognition that he had hypertension, for which he was now receiving treatment. A follow-up treadmill test was also satisfactory, and an angiogram showed only very mild evidence of heart disease, insufficient to explain his symptoms. There was no clear answer for his chest pain, but he was left feeling increasingly worried and perplexed.

For the previous month he had been experiencing dizzy spells and chest pain, which he concluded was almost certainly due to heart disease. He purchased a blood pressure machine which he carried with him at all times, monitoring his blood pressure whenever his symptoms reappeared, keeping it to hand, in his drawer, when he was at work. His GP had already referred him back to the cardiologist, who had reassured him, saying his chest pain was almost certainly non-cardiac, but recognising that John seemed anxious, he had referred him for psychological intervention, which John had reluctantly accepted.

The visit to the cardiologist had really alarmed John, and he did not feel reassured at all. All he could really remember of the visit was that the specialist had said he was only almost certain the pain was not due to heart disease, and John was disappointed that more tests had not been arranged and that the consultant had failed to admit him to hospital for further monitoring. He insisted that he was worried because of the pain, and if that this could be properly explained and dealt with appropriately he would be fine.

The therapist agreed that the pain was causing a great deal of concern, and so asked John to keep a diary of his activities throughout the week, particularly recording when he got any symptoms and whenever he needed to check his blood pressure. He also asked him to record his levels of anxiety every day. John agreed to the diary, although he could not promise to do it all the time as he was under a lot of pressure at work (a comment which the therapist made special note of).

John's completed diary is reproduced in Table 5.1.

John was pleased to have completed the diary, but was worried by the frequency of the pain. He had not noticed any particular pattern as to when it occurred, but was alarmed that the symptoms seemed to appear most days. The therapist began by picking out the highest anxiety scores. These were understandably associated with episodes of pain, but on closer examination it became clear that they were also associated with pressures at work. Moreover, it was noted that intense physical activity, such as pushing a full trolley around the supermarket, shifting a heavy wardrobe across the bedroom and a long

Table 5.1   John's diary of chest pain

Rate anxiety on a score of 0–100, where 0=no anxiety and 100=worst possible anxiety

Wednesday	Thursday	Friday	Saturday	Sunday	Monday	Tuesday
Lunchtime **dizzy**, checked BP, **60**	Meeting cancelled	Bit **dizzy** in morning following a dispute over order, **80**	Supermarket shopping then moved furniture around in daughter's bedroom		**Chest pain** on and off for most of the morning, a bit **breathless, 10** BP checked a few times, **90, tingling**	OK all day really and the order came in on time and was all correct,
Chest pain at 6pm, couldn't face supper, felt sick, **80**, **tingling**	OK all day	**Chest pain** at lunchtime, thought I might have to go home, BP OK, **80**	Gardening, finished off new vegetable patch, **0**	**Dizzy** after gardening, irritable for rest of the day and difficulty sleeping	Still a bit **dizzy**, tired, sorting out issues from meeting, BP OK, **60**	

BP, blood pressure. Text in bold as marked by the therapist.

period of heavy digging in the garden, activities one might normally expect to bring on an episode of angina, were free from pain, dizziness and tingling.

These periods of heavy activity, free from the pressures of work, were also free from anxiety, and John was asked to consider whether the pains and dizziness he had experienced might have been caused by anxiety rather than heart disease. This was revelatory to him and he spontaneously began to divulge how unhappy he was in his new role at the factory. Further evidence that his chest pains were associated with anxiety was provided by applying the Beck Anxiety Inventory (BAI), where it became clear that when he had the pain, he scored very highly for other symptoms of anxiety too. As the work issues were addressed in therapy, and John was persuaded to put his blood pressure machine in the attic, his confidence grew and his chest pains disappeared.

Techniques addressing safety-seeking behaviours

Dealing with checking behaviours

Health-anxious patients frequently check their bodies for signs of disease. This can be for several reasons:

- to look for evidence of new disease
- to monitor an existing perceived problem
- to ward off new disease.

Checking can often be revealed during construction of the formulation, but you may need to ask about it directly (e.g. asking patients whether they check their pulse during an episode of chest pain). It may be identified after you have completed the formulation, and in this case it is important to go back to this, with the patient, and add it in. Patients are sometimes unaware that they check, or that feeling for their pulse constitutes that kind of activity, considering it 'normal' behaviour, for example, when they experience pain. For some patients, checking or generally monitoring their bodies has become a habit and they have to be reminded that they do it.

Sometimes patients check in very subtle ways. A gamekeeper who, following a heart attack, had become health anxious with panic attacks had responded well to initial management where one of the issues addressed was the frequency with which he checked his pulse and felt his heart, to see whether it was still working normally. Despite this improvement, mainly reflected in a cognitive shift from worrying about his heart to worrying (much less) about his anxiety, he still had times in the evenings when he felt tense and hot, which was very unpleasant. After careful questioning it transpired that when out and about on the estate and feeling well, towards the end of the day he would stop and reflect on this and run through a checklist in his mind, mentally ticking off the anxiety symptoms that were absent. After stopping this process, his residual anxiety symptoms quickly settled down.

It can be helpful to ask patients directly for the ways in which they may check their health, as these are often multiple. Some common examples are:

- checking pulse for regularity, strength and speed of heart rate, to make sure their heart is still beating or for missed beats
- checking sputum for colour (equating green sputum with infection) or looking for blood
- checking urine for colour or blood, and often in the case of health professionals, testing it repeatedly with dipstix
- checking stools for consistency and blood
- checking for abdominal tenderness, swelling or lumps, usually by frequent prodding, feeling their 'liver' for evidence of cancer spread
- repeatedly looking in the mirror for changes in appearance or lumps on their tongue or in their throat
- checking the skin for 'moles', marks or general discolouration
- checking breasts for lumps
- examining neck, groin, axillae, etc. for evidence of enlarged glands
- comparing one side of the body with the other looking for discrepancies (patients are often unaware that no person has a completely symmetrical body).

The problem with checking is that it focuses attention on the problem, invariably making it worse. Patients should not be told this, but invited to consider this for themselves and test it out. This can begin within the therapy session. For example, if the symptom is difficulty in swallowing, the exercise of deliberately swallowing 7 times in succession by the patient and therapist together shows this can create discomfort, as can repeatedly prodding the abdomen to see whether there is a lump, if the patient has this concern. Ask your patient what would happen if they repeatedly examined and prodded a part of their body. This should elicit the response that it might make the area more red or uncomfortable, then ask whether there might have been occasions when this had occurred.

This may well lead back to the formulation and the possibility that checking might be one of the factors fuelling the circle of fear, and that modifying this particular behaviour could be a way of breaking out of the circle; in other words, is the checking helping, or is it making things worse? The patient can then be asked to test this out, leading to one of your first behavioural experiments.

Invite the patient to monitor for themselves the effects of checking for their specific problem. This usually takes the form of them finding out what happens to their anxiety levels on days when they check repeatedly, at regular intervals throughout the day, compared with their anxiety on days when they resist checking. The checking can be done on alternate days, but is perhaps best arranged so that they check for two days and then resist for the rest of the week, so that they can test further any cumulative effects over time, which may result from modifying this behaviour.

They are asked to record their anxiety levels at regular specified intervals throughout the day, rating their anxiety on a score of 0–100 (see a template for monitoring anxiety levels in Table 5.2).

Some patients find it difficult to rate anxiety, so it is important to make sure they understand. You may need to get them to identify examples from their previous experience, asking for times when they have been extremely anxious and moderately anxious, and settling on scores for these occasions. These then provide benchmarks against which the patient can measure

Table 5.2   Template for monitoring the effects of checking

For each day, at the times specified, please record your level of anxiety on a scale of 0–100, where 0 = no anxiety, 100 = the worst possible anxiety you could experience

	Checked		No checking				
Time of day	Tue	Wed	Thu	Fri	Sat	Sun	Mon
Morning (first thing)							
Mid-morning							
Lunchtime							
Mid-afternoon							
Teatime							
Bedtime							

future anxiety; you could also record their anxiety for the day you are seeing them, on the sheet, to get them started.

You may also need to ease them into this exercise by offering to take responsibility for ceasing to check, as explained in Box 5.2 (p. 50); they can then be gradually weaned off this as before.

Patients should also be encouraged to include comments on the form (such as 'forgot and checked'), or perhaps that they need to add a new problem, such as 'developed a sore throat', or something unrelated that had upset them. Comments such as these can help interpret the ratings.

In a straightforward, uncomplicated case you would expect to find higher scores on the days when checking took place, then a gradual progressive fall in scores over subsequent days when the checking ceased, as shown in Table 5.3. In such cases, the patient is invited to comment, getting feedback from the form about how helpful, or not, checking is, illustrating that, over time, there is a clear demonstration that stopping checking is helpful.

Sometimes there does not seem to be a pattern on initial inspection. There may be a host of explanations for this; the patient may have continued to check, some other event may have occurred complicating the picture, they may have failed to understand the assignment, and so on. Comments recorded on the form are particularly helpful in these situations and it would be very unusual not to find an underlying pattern after careful

Table 5.3 Example of checking modification experiment I, patient with fear of skin cancer

For each day, at the times specified, please record your level of anxiety on a scale of 0–100, where 0 = no anxiety, 100 = the worst possible anxiety you could experience

	Checked		No checking				
Time of day	Tue	Wed	Thu	Fri	Sat	Sun	Mon
Morning (first thing)	60	70, spot still there	60	50	40	20	20
Mid-morning	60	70	60	40	30	10	Forgot
Lunchtime	60	70	Forgot and checked	40	Forgot	10	Forgot
Mid-afternoon	70, noticed spot	80, mark bigger	60	40	30	10	
Teatime	80	90	50	50	30	20	20
Bedtime	80, couldn't sleep	80	50	50	50	30	20

examination of the list. An example of this is given in Table 5.4. This patient had a fear of a brain tumour and other forms of cancer and would check their body repeatedly for signs of this.

In Table 5.4, clusters of high scores coincided with the development of a cold, and then were maintained by an episode of stomach pain as a consequence of reinstating checking, whereas a cluster of low scores on a checking day corresponded to the visit of the patient's granddaughter when the patient was distracted from her fears. Identification and discussion of these proved quite enlightening and led to this patient being able to cease checking permanently, with a corresponding, and recognised, reduction in anxiety. Once it has been identified that checking is unhelpful it should not be reinstated.

Patients can also check in other ways. One very common way is by searching for information about their particular fears on the internet. Less common now is the use of medical texts, but this does still occur, as does the accumulation and perusal of medical leaflets, and seeking out articles in the media. These sources often give conflicting opinions, leading to

Table 5.4 Example of checking modification experiment II, patient with fear of cancer

For each day, at the times specified, please record your level of anxiety on a scale of 0–100, where 0 = no anxiety, 100 = the worst possible anxiety you could experience

Time of day	Checked		No checking				
	Tue	Wed	Thu	Fri	Sat	Sun	Mon
Morning (first thing)	70	60	40	**60, snuffly, checked**	40	50	50
Mid-morning	80	40, grand-daughter came	30	**60**	20	30	40, pain better, forgot
Lunchtime	80	Forgot	Forgot and checked	**60**	20	30	Forgot
Mid-afternoon	60	30	70	**60, checked**	20	60, stomach ache again, checked	**Pain still there a bit, checked**
Teatime	60	30	40	50	50, stomach ache	**80**	**80**
Bedtime	80	40	**60, nose blocked, checked**	50	**60, felt stomach, sore**	**90, pain still there**	**90, checked, cancer?**

Text in bold as marked by the therapist.

further information-seeking to get at 'the truth', and of course searching on the internet is a particular minefield with its never-ending links to things more serious or potentially disfiguring and at worst, fatal. There are also 'addictive chat rooms' where patients can share their experiences, and although many people can find this helpful, they invariable fuel the fears of those with health anxiety. This form of checking must always be asked about directly as it is increasingly common, and patients should be encouraged to cease this activity early in treatment (by testing out its usefulness as with body-checking outlined earlier, pp. 43–44). A long-term goal of therapy, and a healthy long-term outcome, would be the ability to use the internet sensibly, resisting the urge to explore worrying links on health. It is sometimes useful to ask people why they need to spend so much time worrying, and to illustrate it by saying, 'Do you spend a lot of time thinking about what you would spend your winnings on if you won the lottery?'. No, most people do not, as they would say the chances of winning a lot of money are too small to bother about this. Exactly the same argument can be used to explain why constant worries about their health are equally unproductive.

Some patients also check for signs of disease in their family or close friends, or sometimes even in people they come into contact with. This is usually as a consequence of fearing that they have an infectious disease such as tuberculosis, or a sexually transmitted disease such as chlamydia. One health-anxious patient was convinced that he had acquired HIV by using a toothbrush belonging to a colleague while on a business trip. He also became increasingly concerned that he had passed on the infection to his wife. He underwent repeated negative testing at the local genitourinary medicine clinic, but was only briefly reassured each time. As well as constantly checking himself for signs of illness, he began to scrutinise his wife for any sign of debilitation that might imply a compromised immune system. This led to him misinterpreting a transitory rash she had developed – actually explained by contact dermatitis from a new body cream – as incontrovertible evidence that he had given her HIV and so had the same disease himself in an advanced form. Once again, the value of this particular form of checking can be tested in the same way as in the examples described earlier.

Dealing with reassurance-seeking

Health-anxious patients repeatedly seek reassurance, but, unlike other patients, they fail to experience any lasting relief from this. Any relief they feel, although very welcome at the time, is short lasting and their fears soon return. Because reassurance usually has immediate benefit, it is reinforced and patients often develop a pattern of repeatedly seeking further reassurance, and so compound the problem.

Patients seek reassurance in many ways; sometimes very openly and obviously, but at other times indirectly or covertly. They may seek reassurance by visiting health professionals (they often have very frequent visits to their GP) or by asking family and friends. They may ask others to check on a particular concern, for example a mark on the skin, or just ask indirectly, for example whether their spouse thinks they are looking well.

The need for repeated reassurance can become very time consuming, lead to a breakdown in relationships with doctors, family and friends and the repetitive nature of it can become counterproductive and pathological in itself, almost like a form of compulsive behaviour in obsessive–compulsive disorder (OCD). Very frequently, the need for reassurance can be included in the formulation, or if subsequently identified, can be added to this later.

The issue of excessive reassurance-seeking is probably best broached two–three sessions into treatment. This will be after the patient has formally engaged, a formulation has been developed and the therapist understands what maintains the patient's health anxiety. The extent to which the patient engages in reassurance-seeking should be gently assessed. These patients often seek reassurance in many different ways.

Discussion should centre on the negative effect of reassurance by its focus on the need to have the constant support of others, rather than the more constructive approach of being able to manage their health concerns themselves. Reassurance-seeking can become a problem behaviour in itself, wasting time and putting a strain on important relationships. It is helpful to ask patients exactly how they feel when they receive reassurance, for how long they feel better, whether and how soon their fears return, and the effect this has on the wish for more reassurance.

You can then invite the patient to try a different approach to see whether the reassurance-seeking is in fact helpful or whether it could be fuelling their fears. This is what such a conversation might look like:

Therapist: It seems to me that al5though you can feel better after you have asked your partner about [complaint] or been to the doctor, it doesn't tend to last very long and you feel the need to go back. So I am wondering just how helpful this reassurance is in the long run. I wonder if we could try a week of not asking for reassurance and see how that makes you feel. Do you think you could try that for me?

Patient: OK. I could try that.

Therapist: Good. I'm now going to write down all the ways you have sought reassurance recently (lists the ways with the patient until full agreement on list). I want you to try to stop each of these behaviours – all of them – until your next appointment. Do you think you can do that?

Patient: I'm not sure about that. What if I get that rash again or my tongue doesn't feel right, or my cough comes back?

Therapist: Well, haven't we already discussed this? You will remember that we have already talked about other ways of managing these sensations or symptoms. For example, you could avoid checking the problem, putting it on a list of symptoms to be checked 10 days later, or the other methods we have discussed. These are new skills that we want to test out and find if they can help your anxiety.

Patient (doubtfully): Well, I could try, I suppose. But it might be difficult; I haven't done it before.

Therapist: Let's see how you get on. I could offer to take responsibility for your symptoms until I see you again. This would help you resist going to the GP about any of your symptoms, trying to avoid asking family or friends about any issues concerning health, or asking for medical second opinions.

This is an important step for the patient, but often quite difficult for them to do. They will need a lot of encouragement and perhaps require a bit of help deciding how they can implement this new behaviour. This can be particularly difficult if they repeatedly ask close family members for reassurance when they are very worried, so they will need to discuss with you how they plan to avoid doing this. They may still go to them and ask for comfort, provided it is not for reassurance. To help them test out these new behaviours they should be encouraged to go back through the work they have done already in terms of formulations, pie charts and listing symptoms. You can also offer to take responsibility for their symptoms; this can be very helpful if they recognise you as having skills in medicine as well as psychology. You can then wean them off gradually over subsequent sessions.

As with other behavioural changes, it is very important that you follow up the results of this at their next therapy session: discussing how difficult it was to implement, how successful they were and how it made them feel (typically, worse at the start but easier as time progressed). It is also important to get a feedback on how, for example, their partner felt about it.

Stopping the need to seek reassurance can be very empowering for patients, and they often feel very proud of themselves as a consequence. It frequently also leads to an increase in self-esteem, as they have often been humiliated by responses they have received in the past, as their family, friends and eventually even primary care services have become increasingly exasperated.

It is important to tease these responses out of the patient, write them down and feed them back with further encouragement and praise. Once they have accomplished this new way of behaving it is important to maintain it.

Techniques to develop new understanding

Dealing with 'noisy bodies'

'Listing symptoms' is a technique that can help those patients with particularly 'noisy bodies', and those who are repeatedly reporting new symptoms.

Health-anxious patients tend to be hypervigilant for, and readily tune into, bodily sensations and changes, often catastrophically interpreting them as further evidence of underlying disease. A summary of a useful strategy for dealing with recurrent symptoms is shown in Box 5.2.

With this technique the patients are not being told to ignore their symptoms, an approach which paradoxically can tend to make them worse (remember, the more you try to suppress an intrusive thought, the more it

---

Box 5.2 Techniques for dealing with recurring symptoms

- Begin by exploring with your patient the difference between symptoms of disease and bodily sensations or changes.
- Weigh up with them how likely it is a doctor would want to see or investigate someone who had only noticed something minor wrong in the past few days.
- Lead on to working out with the patient a reasonable length of time something would need to be present before medical attention/reassurance needed to be sought. For health-anxious patients, this might be negotiated to a week or 10 days.
- Suggest the patient might test this out for themselves, which can then lead up to presenting the idea that the next time they notice something wrong, they could make a note in their diary or on a list and then see whether it is still there a week later (invariably, it won't be, or the patient will be less bothered by it).
- If this seems too threatening for them, offer to take responsibility for the symptom, initially taking full responsibility, then as they progress, gradually reducing the level of responsibility, maybe to 75% by the next visit, 50% by the next and so on until they are bearing the load themselves.
- Gradually, the patient should be able to put things on the list without telling you what they are, or even that they have done it, and eventually they should be able to do it in their head, or rarely feel the need to do it.
- Finally, they will come to realise that most of these bodily changes do not constitute a threat.

---

springs to mind). Instead they are learning, by testing it out for themselves, a new way of managing the problem, which can lead to a more realistic interpretation of bodily sensations, 'symptoms' and changes.

Conducting surveys

Patients with high health anxiety tend to overestimate the likelihood of developing an illness. They feel it is 'only a matter of time' before they become unwell, or, if other family members develop problems, believe that means there is an increased risk in the family that will extend to them. Sometimes, they feel they are 'jinxed' in some way, or bring bad luck, and that people who come into contact with them will become ill, or that everyone around them seems to be ill. Mostly this is because those with high health anxiety tend to selectively attend to information they hear about others who are ill and ignore or discount those around them who are well. Surveys can be useful in these cases, helping to normalise the patient's situation.

Surveys can be done both by the patient and their therapist, effectively doubling the information obtained. They can contain information directly from the patient's own experience or they can involve asking others. Patients who claim everyone they know is ill, or dying of cancer, are asked how many people they know in their street, and how many are ill. Likewise, they are asked to consider the same problem for everyone employed where they work, their children's school friends, families, their extended family, and friends. They are then asked of those who are ill, how many have recently become ill, or are these ongoing problems, how much can be accounted for by age (e.g. increased risk of infections in schoolchildren and malignancy and heart disease in the elderly), and how many had an increased risk, for example, being heavy smokers or grossly overweight. They are then invited to consider how many are doing well or recovering with treatment. The therapist can then do the exercise themselves with the patient and they can compare experiences. What they tend to find is that their experiences are comparable, that the proportion of those they know who are ill is in fact less than they had assumed, and that much was accounted for by factors such as age and lifestyle. The survey can be extended to asking others in the patient's environment to do the same exercise and compare their findings with those of the patient (Case example 5.4).

Case example 5.4: Anxiety about many diseases

Patricia had had generalised anxiety and high health anxiety for years. Convinced that she was developing Parkinson's disease or, at the very least, dementia, she also had underlying worries about cancer, and was convinced that she almost invited ill health as 'everybody' around her was ill. Recently, her stepfather had developed a chronic form of leukaemia, and then her father was found to have terminal lung cancer. In addition, her daughter, who had recently started nursery, had had repeated upper respiratory infections, and on one occasion a nasty chest infection that had required antibiotics, to which she had been found to be allergic, requiring a trip to the accident and emergency department. A work colleague of her husband's had also recently had a stroke, which was, however, due to a recognised treatable underlying cause and he was making an excellent recovery.

Patricia was asked to name as many people as she could in the street where she lived and the surrounding neighbourhood, house by house. Although she did not know everybody personally, she knew quite a lot of them well, and was able to supply a fair amount of information about the rest. She surprised herself by how much detail she could recall, spontaneously concluding that her memory was not as bad as she had thought! Not only that, but she was able to report that as far as she knew, they were nearly all well. There were some elderly folk who struggled to get about, and one man who had chronic severe breathing problems, also two children up the road had recently been off school with chickenpox, but otherwise they seemed a pretty healthy bunch. The therapist then performed the same exercise for her experience. To their joint amusement, her recall was a little less good, but the conclusions were similar.

Patricia was also asked to consider that both her stepfather and her natural father were elderly, and had previously experienced good health. The former was expected to have a normal lifespan with treatment, and her father's development of cancer could be entirely explained by having a history of lifelong heavy smoking. She was able to conclude that attending nursery school exposed children to a lot of infections, and that drug allergies were commonplace. Another survey revealed how frequent they were, so 'normalising' this particular event, and the fact that neither the patient nor the therapist had ever known anyone personally who had died from a drug allergy, served to reduce Patricia's concern further.

Surveys of personal experience such as these show how the patient's perception of the incidence of ill health can become distorted. This conclusion can be cemented by the realisation that it is also possible to overestimate illness via the media, as they frequently highlight medical catastrophes and mistakes, because they are not typical and are thus 'newsworthy'. How many reports are there of commonplace illnesses from which patients recover quickly, or how there has not been much illness about? Would these be 'headline-grabbers' and would anybody bother to read them?

Linking medically unexplained symptoms to anxiety using the Beck Anxiety Inventory

Linking medically unexplained symptoms to anxiety is primarily done by the diary technique (see pp. 40–42), but further supporting evidence can be obtained by the use of the Beck Anxiety Inventory (Table 5.5; Beck *et al*, 1988), or indeed any other anxiety-rating scale. This inventory lists common symptoms and feelings associated with anxiety on a scale of severity.

The patient is asked to remember when they were last experiencing an unpleasant episode of their particularly troublesome symptom and to record whether they were experiencing any other of the problems listed in the scale, noting whether each one was present and to what extent. The form is initially presented to the patient with the top folded over so that they are unaware that they are filling out a scale that is designed to measure anxiety, and of course they are completing it with reference to a specific event, not over the preceding week as the form states.

It is highly likely that many of the items will be represented in the moderate or severe columns and this cluster can be highlighted. Discussion can then take place that whatever else was going on regarding the particular symptom that had concerned the patient at the time, they were also highly anxious. This can also show that associated symptoms that were also present at the time and are included on the list, such as dizziness, are not necessarily medically associated with the main symptom, for example, headache or non-cardiac chest pain, but a consequence of related anxiety. Once again this opens the door to a less threatening explanation for all the symptoms.

Completing a standardised measure which lists a series of troublesome symptoms and experiences that are recognised to coexist can be a tangible relief for these patients. Not only does it help provide the link with anxiety, it also helps the patient feel understood and less alone with their fear.

As this scale measures severity, it can also be used to measure improvement as therapy progresses.

Behavioural experiments

Behavioural experiments broadly take two forms: information-gathering experiments such as monitoring the effects of checking or not checking

Table 5.5 Beck Anxiety Inventory, adapted

Name			Date	

Below is a list of common symptoms of anxiety. Indicate how much you have been bothered by each symptom during the past week, including today. Please carefully rate each item in the list, by placing an X in the corresponding space in the column next to each symptom.

Symptom	Not at all	Mildly (It did not bother me much)	Moderately (It was very unpleasant, but I could stand it)	Severely (I could barely stand it)
1 Numbness or tingling				
2 Feeling hot				
3 Wobbliness in legs				
4 Unable to relax				
5 Fear of the worst happening				
6 Dizzy or light-headed				
7 Heart pounding or racing				
8 Unsteady				
9 Terrified				
10 Nervous				
11 Feelings of choking				
12 Hands trembling				
13 Shaky				
14 Fear of losing control				
15 Difficulty breathing				
16 Fear of dying				
17 Scared				

the body, and asking patients to test out their new less threatening beliefs as therapy progresses. Patients with health anxiety often set up patterns of avoidant behaviour. This may be to minimise further risk or deterioration to their health, or because they are avoiding an activity that has made them feel worse in the past. They may feel that they had a lucky escape once before and must therefore avoid taking that risk again. Avoiding exercise is a frequent example. A typical case might be where an episode of more strenuous activity had brought on (normal) palpitations that were misinterpreted as the sign of an impending heart attack; immediate cessation of activity relieved the symptoms, reinforcing the belief that by avoiding activity in the future and resting, the person could avoid running that risk again. As a consequence, they became less fit, and as their exercise tolerance dropped this was further misinterpreted as progression of disease, and thus it became even more important not to 'overdo it'.

Sometimes patients consider themselves so ill that they see little point in pursuing any form of normal activity, becoming increasingly isolated and depressed. In cases when therapy has revealed alternative, less threatening explanation for their worrying symptoms, the next stage is directed towards enabling the patient to see how these problematic behaviours have developed and test their validity by behavioural experiments (Case example 5.5).

Case example 5.5: Fear of sudden death

Naomi had developed high health anxiety after the death of her mother. They had both worked at the local hospital; Naomi in reception and her mother a volunteer at the hospital shop. Naomi's mother had collapsed at work 9 months previously and despite receiving fairly immediate attention, resuscitation was unsuccessful. She was taken to the mortuary where a post-mortem showed she had had a massive stroke caused by a vascular abnormality in the brain. Naomi was devastated by her mother's sudden death and terrified that she would suffer the same fate. She developed headaches, noticed trembling in her little finger when she was using the keyboard, and felt dizzy at times, as if she might collapse. Her diary recorded that her symptoms were worse when she was at work, and particularly marked on the days when she worked on the out-patient clinic which was quite near the shop. Naomi had avoided walking past the shop since her mother had died, taking a longer route, around the outside of the hospital, to the out-patients department. She told her colleagues that she liked to get some fresh air. She also avoided walking past the mortuary department, and got off the bus a stop earlier, walking a longer distance to bypass it. Even if she had to walk in that direction in the hospital, she felt it might mean she would die and be taken there.

The diary had established that there was a possible link between her medically unexplained symptoms and anxiety, and through the use of the Beck equation (see Chapter 2), Naomi was building evidence that it was highly unlikely that she would experience the same fate as her mother. She was then asked to consider the fact that everyone had to die some time and that if they died in hospital they would be taken to the mortuary. With her therapist, they conducted separate surveys of the people they knew where a relative or friend had undergone a post-mortem, and they both reached the conclusion that it was fairly common, and in many cases a 'matter of fact'. It was also clear that her mother was no longer in the mortuary and many other people had passed through there since. Naomi began to lose the images of her mother lying dead on the floor, and replace them with memories of the fun times they had had together.

The next stage of the therapy was exposure to the hospital shop and the mortuary. Naomi was encouraged initially to walk past the shop on her way to the clinic. She was prepared for this by the discussion that it would probably be staffed by different people now. When she tried this, it was easier than she expected, and she bumped into an old friend on the way. The next stage was buying something from the shop. It was an old colleague of her mum who served her, and they had a chat about how things were going. When asked how she felt after this, she was surprised to find that she had experienced hardly any symptoms, and in fact felt comforted. Walking past the mortuary had seemed an impossible feat to start with, but she felt emboldened by her other success and managed it with ease. She no longer got off the bus a stop too soon. Gradually, her symptoms disappeared and her anxiety diminished. She began to make plans for the future, and booked a holiday abroad, something she had been completely unable to do before.

Testing out new beliefs in this way is the next crucial step in challenging fear, and by putting beliefs into practice cements them in place.

Developing a shared understanding between patient and therapist: helping the patient choose to change

Fear of disease rather than disease attribution

This technique is designed to help the patient recognise that their underlying problem is fear of *anxiety* about having or developing a particular disease rather than fear of *actually having* or being about to develop the disease itself.

The construction of the vicious circle/flower and other techniques is intended to highlight the anxiety generated by their fear/conviction of disease, with all the negative connotations this evokes.

Helping the patient generate the case for fear of having a particular disease, rather than actually having it, allows an important cognitive shift. The patient is asked to consider two alternative explanations for their health anxiety, and list the advantages of each. If they have already progressed in therapy you can make the case for the evidence for these two hypotheses, as in the example in Table 5.6.

This can then be built on as a framework, encouraging patients to add further evidence for the 'fear of' hypothesis as the therapy continues.

This can further be backed up by asking whether there have ever been occasions when something has turned out better than the person thought it would, and getting them to generate examples of this, including examples that are not health related. Sometimes, this can usefully be done as homework. These examples can then be examined in more detail asking the question whether, in retrospect, their anticipatory anxiety had in fact been helpful or altered the outcome. This is an important issue to address, as often health-anxious people feel that they need to worry to protect themselves from future harm.

Counting the cost of health anxiety

Living with health anxiety and consequent dysfunctional beliefs has a cost. With the patient, you can examine this by looking at how this affects their way of life, identifying the restrictions it places on them and the things it stops them from doing, how it affects their relationships and their mood, and the difficulties experienced in living with this fear. Sum all these up and then ask the patient the advantages of doing something about the fear. This works best when the costs can be worked up into a fairly long list. For some patients, their 'illness' (and of course there may be a confirmed medical

Table 5.6 Illness and fear of illness explanations for patients' symptoms

'I have brain cancer'	'I have fear of brain cancer'
The therapist asks:	*And:*
'What would be the advantages of having brain cancer?'	'What would be the advantages of this being *fear* of having brain cancer (but you don't actually have it)?'
Typical responses might be:	
'None'	*Typical responses might be:*
or	• 'I wouldn't have brain cancer'
'I'd have an answer and they could start treating it… but I don't want to have it.'	• 'I wouldn't have to have those horrible treatments'
	• 'I'm not going to die'
	• 'I will be able to see my children grow up'
	• 'If it is fear, can I get treatment for this?' *(To which the response would be: 'Yes, this is how the CBT works')*
The therapist then asks:	*Or, more excitingly:*
'Can we build up any evidence for this actually being cancer?'	'Can we build up any evidence for this being *fear* of cancer as opposed to actually having the disease?'
Here the patient might say:	*Here you start drawing on evidence from the work done so far, for example the conclusions derived from the pie charts, the pyramid, the effects of stopping checking, the association of headache with other symptoms of anxiety and the fact that they occur in stressful situations. Together, these will have generated alternative, less threatening explanations for their headache, and so they are listed in this column, supporting evidence for the 'fear of brain cancer' model. As the evidence stacks up in this column the patient can begin to see real evidence generated from themselves (in collaboration with their therapist) that they may not have the disease that they fear.*
'Well, my headaches have been present for 2 years, they are persistent.'	
You could then discuss the facts that, for instance: recently the headaches have been a bit better after the patient stopped checking; if the patient had had headaches for 2 years due to a brain tumour they might be more ill; recently the patient had noticed that the headaches came on when they were worried about various things. This develops a rationale for including 'persistent headaches' in the 'fear of' list and duly moving it over to the other column.	

condition underlying it, compounded by health anxiety) has become so all-encompassing that they may have forgotten what it was to feel 'normal' and they may require help to tease out what has become missing from their life. The list should be comprehensive, covering day-to-day activities, including work and home life, family issues, leisure time and holidays, their relationships and friendships, including their social life, and their overall sense of worth, including what they are or were able to offer others.

You are jointly looking at their general quality of life now compared with before they became ill, or for those in whom health anxiety has been a very long-term problem, compared with what might have been. This is then summarised for the patient and discussed. This should then lead on to an exploration of how the patient would like to live their life, what would they like to be able to do, and how would they like to be remembered?

Thinking errors

People with health anxiety experience distress because they think in particularly negative ways. Negative thinking can make you feel anxious, depressed, angry, or any combination of these. Errors in thinking, some already identified in earlier chapters, together with maladaptive behaviour patterns are very important in health anxiety. This is because they maintain the fears and worries about ill health, despite all the other evidence that there is nothing physically wrong. Working through these errors gradually with your patient, finding examples from their own experience, can be very helpful. Often homework can entail the patient identifying these errors themselves. The error box (Box 5.3) summarises many of these.

Other examples of thinking errors include:

- 'Everything always goes wrong for me in April, I'm more likely to get ill in that month.'
- 'I have had problems in my right arm and my right leg. This is a sign of weakness in that side and means I will get further trouble.'

For example, an anxious person might notice the sensation of pins and needles in their arm and on looking up this symptom on the internet, finds through various links that it can be a symptom of multiple sclerosis, but of course there are many other causes – such as lying in a certain position. Other errors (Box 5.4) compound those in Box 5.3.

All these types of thoughts make people feel that their health is under threat. The errors in thought are often hard to recognise at first, because they have happened so often, coming into the mind automatically, like a habit. These thoughts have some other characteristics:

- they are unreasonable, and the aim of therapy is learning to challenge them with more logical thoughts
- even though the thoughts are not true, they *seem* completely sensible, especially when patients are very worried about their health
- these thoughts serve no useful function and can interfere with progress if they are not recognised as dysfunctional; they almost always generate anxiety.

Once the patient has begun to identify the thinking errors, they can start the exercise of cognitive restructuring. Alternative, more rational ways of thinking can be considered. Once they have mastered this exercise they are more ready to accept the less threatening alternative and this helps them challenge the original beliefs and behaviours.

Rituals are sometimes present and often occur as a consequence of superstitious thinking. We all do this to some extent – 'touching wood' to 'prevent' harm is probably the most common example. In patients with health anxiety there are countless other examples, such as repeated counting and relying on 'lucky numbers', having objects in exactly the same place at all times, cleaning in exactly the same order and many, many others. Logically, such things cannot affect our health. They tend to keep attention on worries and help to maintain the whole problem. Therapy is directed at resisting such behaviours while measuring the effects of this resistance on anxiety over time. Initially, the patient feels very anxious, but this subsides gradually, and if this resistance is maintained, the need to perform the particular ritual diminishes, freeing the patient up to live a more normal existence.

Box 5.3 Thinking errors, part I

- **Jumping to conclusions** When a symptom is noticed, the person with health anxiety immediately thinks that this means illness, without stopping to weigh up any other possible causes, for example: 'This pain is so bad that it must mean I am ill'; 'I'm sweating more than I should in this hot spell, I must be ill'.
- **Catastrophising** This is jumping to the worst conclusion. So the person will not just think that they have an illness, but will assume that the illness is a very serious, or even fatal, condition. They may start to imagine all sorts of unpleasant consequences, in terms of severe pain and suffering and also in terms of distress to family and friends. This type of thinking often goes further into anticipating the outcome of treatment for an illness, so the person will often assume that if they did have a condition, it would be impossible to cure, believing, for example: 'This must be cancer, and from now on I will be just a burden to my family; 'Despite what they say, no one is ever really cured of cancer'.
- **Superstitious thinking** Some patients believe that worrying about their health somehow protects them from any harm, concluding, 'If I think I am well I will tempt fate'. Many people also feel that as everyone develops an illness at some time, the fact that they have been well for a while means that the time must come for them to develop a serious illness.
- **Overgeneralising** This is a very common error. If someone hears about an illness or symptoms, they may assume from any similarities or common factors that they have the same illness themselves. This can take curious forms, for example, if a celebrity of the same age as the patient has just developed cancer, it somehow makes it more likely that the patient will develop cancer too.
- **Making false links** It is easy to get hold of the wrong information about health, accentuated recently by various sources, for instance the internet, and to incorrectly assume that certain symptoms are always linked with illnesses. A man who was convinced, despite negative tests, that he had the infection, chlamydia, felt that this diagnosis was incontrovertible when his wife developed toothache. He assumed this was because her immune system was so damaged by the infection that she was getting other infections.

Flow diagram of choice of technique

The initial assessment has been outlined in Chapter 4. To help clarify the next stages, use can be made of a flow diagram (Fig. 5.3). Yet this is only a guide; as you become more experienced, specific techniques will spring to mind as being appropriate for the situation encountered at the time.

Box 5.4 Thinking errors, part II

- **Ignoring the positive** It is easy to assume that an illness is present, while ignoring signs of good health. Listing evidence of good health which can be incorporated into the table of fear of disease can be a very useful exercise.
- **Exaggerating** Here the error is to overestimate the chances of coming down with a particular illness: 'I look like my sister who had heart trouble, that must mean that I have it as well'.
- **Selective attention and memory** When someone is worried about an illness, they often only tend to notice and remember information which fits in with their worries. All this information then serves to make them more convinced that they are ill.
- **All or nothing** It is a common error to think that the body can only be either entirely free from symptoms or physically ill. Another example of this is the view that both sides of the body have to be identical and if there is the slightest variation this is interpreted as a sign of illness.
- **Thinking in certainties** Another error that the health anxious patient makes is to strive for the certainty that he or she is perfectly well. Clearly no one can ever be completely certain that they are not going to develop an illness, in the same way that you cannot be completely certain that you will not be run over some time in the future. Patients with health anxiety often need help with dealing with uncertainty, and say things such as, 'I must always know that I am completely well, I had a test 3 months ago, maybe it has "run out" and I am due for another'.
- **Preoccupation with health** Very little time is spent thinking of anything else.
- **Misunderstanding medical information** This is extremely common, especially as medicine becomes more complicated and technical. It is hardly surprising that people who have not had any medical training may not have fully understood the information they have been given, especially if consultations are rushed. They often feel they have not been given a proper explanation for their symptoms and so do not feel reassured, making comments such as, 'The doctor cannot be sure I am well without doing tests or an operation to look inside me', and 'He said that special blood cells have caused my allergy, but I have read that special blood cells cause cancer'.
- **Responsibility for health** The patient believes it important to continually monitor their own health, otherwise there is a danger that a problem will be missed at an early stage and then prove difficult to treat. They would never be able to forgive themselves for being so irresponsible.

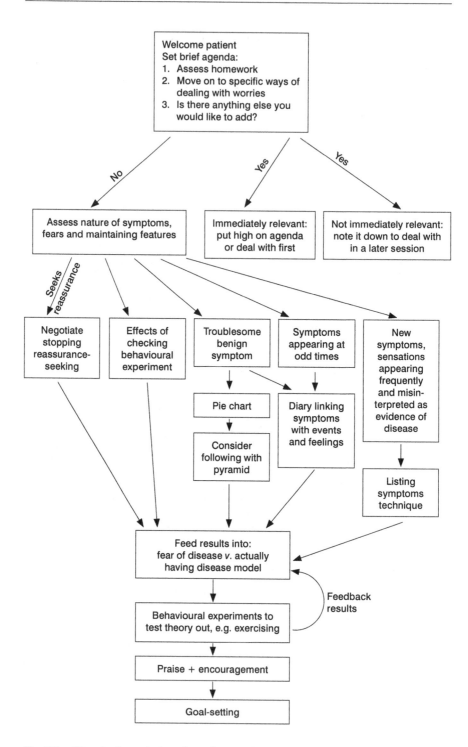

Fig. 5.3 After the formulation: flow diagram for choice of technique.

Chapter messages

- Be prepared to use pie charts and pyramids whenever the interpretation of a symptom has been magnified inappropriately.
- Remember to allow the patient to select the proportions for each pie chart and pyramid; this is a collaborative effort and the final result constitutes their own judgement.
- Identify which symptoms may be more likely to be due to anxiety than physical disease; these can often be identified using the diary technique.
- Most health-anxious patients check too much and always look for evidence of their suspicions, as it reinforces anxiety.
- Getting the patient to recognise that 'fear of disease' is their main problem rather than 'actual disease' can be a breakthrough in treatment.
- Thinking errors and reassurance reinforce health anxiety and always need attention in treatment.

CHAPTER 6

Homework:
setting and evaluation

The rationale for homework

Homework is an integral part of CBT and is normally introduced from the start of therapy. Initially, it takes the form of going over the work done in the session, looking through any written material, and importantly, listening to the recording of the session, which means that ideally all sessions should be recorded. This is not essential but is a very good form of homework, particularly if patients have been very anxious in the session and not able to concentrate well. Some patients feel awkward or embarrassed listening to themselves talking about their problems, or may find it difficult finding the time, or initially be reluctant to listen to the recording, particularly if they want to listen to it alone. Nevertheless, this should always be encouraged. Hearing themselves talking about their problems can be revelatory for some patients, and as, in effect, you are going through the session again, much more information is retained. While listening to and going over any new recorded or written information remains continuous during therapy, the next phase of homework is usually an information-gathering exercise. For example, the patient may be asked to record anxiety levels at regular intervals throughout the day, while recording their activity at the time, to attempt to identify a pattern in their distress, or, typically, to evaluate the effects of checking and not checking on their health. Later on in therapy, homework is devised to test out new, alternative hypotheses that have been developed, providing first-hand experience for the patient, thereby helping to build up a body of evidence for the new hypothesis.

Throughout this handbook various examples of homework have been given, but in this section I cover how to approach the setting of this task, how to evaluate it and what to do if it does not go to plan.

Approaching the setting of homework

The homework should be relevant, purposeful and derived from what has been discussed within the therapy session, and the therapist should stress this association. For example:

Therapist: You have been telling me about some particularly distressing episodes of acute anxiety over the past 2 weeks. I think in the course of this we have established that you have been very worried for almost all of that time. I wonder if we could look at the possibility of you keeping a diary of how you feel during the next week and bring it with you at your next visit. How does that sound?

Patient: I suppose I could do that, but as I've said and you've repeated, I worry all the time.

It is then important to explain directly the point of the homework, and why it is useful, but without anticipating the findings:

Therapist: It would be helpful to know if there was any pattern to the extent to which you worry, to see if there were times when it was particularly bad, so that we can get a real 'fingerprint' of your anxiety.

Patient: I can try, but I've never been much good at this, and I could really tell you right now what the answer will be – it'll be terrible all the time!

Here, the therapist is trying to see whether there is a fluctuation in the patient's anxiety, as the patient has said they worry all the time and it is always severe (although, in practice, this is rarely the case). Finding fluctuations and their associations is helpful for guiding future therapy, and, in addition, it helps patients become more in touch with sensations and other feelings going on in their bodies.

If, during the session, homework around the topic seems important, but you are unsure how to construct it, leave it until the next session when you have had a chance to work it out properly. You can indicate that you will be discussing this within the next session; meanwhile, the patient can concentrate on listening to the recording of what you have just been working on. If you are unclear about what you are asking for in terms of homework you can be sure the patient will be unclear as well.

It is then crucial to explain simply and carefully exactly what you wish the patient to do:

Therapist: Good, I'm glad you feel able to give it a try, now what I would like you to do is...

Repeat the instructions and ask the patient whether they understand and feel they would be able to attempt it. Listen and observe carefully how they respond. If they seem hesitant, reflect this back:

Therapist: I get the feeling that you are a bit unsure about this. Do you feel this is going to be a problem?

If they seem unable to explain the reason for their hesitancy, suggest some reasons why this might be a problem, never forgetting that some people have difficulty reading and writing – the last time they did homework they were probably at school and are far from well-disposed towards it. You can list these possible reasons and look at them together; some may be dismissed immediately, others may be added, but it allows a framework for discussion, validating the patient's fears. Some general examples of these are:

- Perhaps you think this will be difficult to do at home?
- Will you find this a problem if other people see what you are doing?
- Do you feel this will be too difficult?
- Do you think it's not really relevant or important?
- Is it a bit unclear?
- Do you have difficulty reading what I have written?
- Is it difficult to read or understand this form?
- Are you worried you might feel worse?
- Are you concerned that something might be missed? (This is usually an issue when you are testing out changes in behaviour such as the effects of a patient checking or monitoring for ill health, introducing times when they do not check.)
- Does this make you feel unsafe?

The homework is likely to be more successfully completed if you can anticipate potential difficulties. For example, some patients, if being asked to complete a chart, may find this embarrassing or inconvenient to do while at work; you could suggest they make a mental note and do it when they get home. Others may need ways to remind themselves to complete a task on a regular basis.

If patients seem unclear about how to fill out a chart, it is a good idea to start doing one together within the session, if possible getting the patient to fill it in.

Before the session is completed ask the patient to explain back to you exactly what it is you want them to do; for example, you might say:

> 'Just to check that I've explained all this properly, I wonder if you could just run through what you think I've asked you to do. Is there anything that's still unclear for any reason?'

The patient should then be encouraged to do their best to attempt the homework, remembering that doing the exercise you have negotiated with them may be a very unfamiliar one, or may involve them testing out something new, involving taking a risk. There may also be unforeseen difficulties, or the patient may have residual uncertainties and you want them to feel able to return even if they were unable to undertake the task. Gentle encouragement is the key, acknowledging that they might find it difficult and they may encounter problems.

Behavioural experiments

With behavioural experiments, where you may be asking the patient to test out something they may associate with risk or feeling unsafe, it is especially important to remember to take very small steps. Your patient will guide you in what they feel these steps might be. If you decide on something too difficult, the patient may either not be able to do it, or they will fail. This is not irretrievable, but it highlights that you have not understood the extent of the patient's fear or properly explored their problem and this will need sensitive re-evaluation. Failure must not be considered the patient's fault.

When the patient is being asked to undertake homework that they associate with risk, you can ease them into it by offering to take responsibility for them. For example, you and your patient might have agreed to test out the effects of increasing the extent to which they exercise or spend time on their own. These may be potentially terrifying situations, for example, if the patient fears they might experience an acute cardiac event with no one there to help. With these two examples, you will have already established where necessary, from the notes or from the responsible medical personnel, that what you are going to test out is safe, and of course you will have explored with the patient the extent to which anxiety is driving their fear and what this is costing them in how it impinges on their life. You can encourage them to undertake the homework by taking full personal responsibility for it, and clearly need to be satisfied in your own mind that it is substantially free of risk. As patients undertake the exercises, over subsequent sessions you can gradually reduce the level of responsibility, eventually leading to them assuming full responsibility for their actions.

Also important to success is alerting the patient to the fact that the task set is *expected* to generate a degree of anxiety, and so they should not be put off by this. Go over again with them through the symptoms of arousal, using the Beck Anxiety Inventory if necessary, helping them anticipate some of the symptoms they may be going to feel. These symptoms are usually mild and transient, but in some patients where this is not explained, and the task set too difficult, they may be severe and prevent the homework being completed.

Sometimes some of the patient's fears can be projected to the therapist, but it is imperative that you do not exhibit your own underlying anxieties regarding the exercise the patient has been asked to undertake. This would completely undermine the exercise, and as a consequence, it would assuredly fail. It is important to realise as a therapist that nothing is ever risk free, but what you are doing with your patient is helping them to learn to manage risk more appropriately.

Evaluation of the work

If you have set homework you must *always* remember to ask about it. If you omit to do this, the patient will be very unlikely to undertake any more. Often patients have completed this work diligently, under difficult circumstances. They may feel worried about showing written homework to you in case they have not done it properly or in case they got it wrong. They may also be puzzled or concerned about the findings, and unforeseen events may have occurred that have made it harder for them to accomplish the task.

Whatever, or however little, the patient has managed to do they must be congratulated on their attempt. Even if they failed to complete any of the tasks set, thank them for considering it and thinking about it, then gently explore with them the difficulties they found. Also explore how they got on. How difficult was it? Were there any particular problems? How did they feel about doing it?

Homework always shows something, even if it is not what you expect to find, so take time to go through it with your patient. Discuss the findings together, remembering that this is their work and you are privileged to see it. Look for patterns to interpret and feed back any findings, helping the patient fit these into work you have already done. A typical example might be that an exercise in resisting repeatedly checking part of the body is found to produce a reduction in anxiety. You can then together go back to the formulation, identify where the checking activity occurred, and see how that particular activity was helping to drive the patient's vicious circle of fear.

You and your patient should both keep a copy of any written homework, as much for encouragement as to refer back to later on in therapy, to show how much the patient has moved on.

With behavioural experiments involving increasing exposure to risk, the next stage is to move forward, gradually increasing the risk, tailoring it more specifically, based on feedback from the patient.

With this aspect of the work you are doing together it is a good opportunity to start incorporating simple goals. Introducing and meeting these fairly early on can bring about an enormous sense of achievement. Often these patients have been living in a constant state of fear, and the sense that they are starting to master it should be instilled as soon as you can.

Encourage the patient to feel proud of what they have achieved.

When homework does not go to plan

There are a variety of reasons why homework does not go to plan:

- it was not relevant
- the patient is not fully engaged in therapy
- it was not explained clearly
- it was not negotiated properly with the patient
- it was too difficult
- it was too complicated
- too much homework was set
- there were unidentified underlying problems with literacy
- lack of motivation (this is not usually a problem in patients with health anxiety unless there is associated depression)
- sabotage by family or friends
- there has been a change in circumstances or unforeseen events have occurred, preventing its completion.

It is important to carefully consider which of these factors may have played a part and address them, remembering that there may well be multiple problems. It is also helpful to acknowledge where the problems were with the patient, particularly as they may feel to blame or that they have failed, or that they will never be able to get better. So being able to say something along the lines of 'I think I (or we) made things much too difficult here as a first step', or admitting that you did not explain things clearly enough, and being open to suggestions from the patient as to why it did not work, will reap dividends for the next attempt.

While discussing this, it is crucial that the lack of homework, or its lack of success, should *not* be labelled as failure; the homework was wrong, not the patient. Endeavour to maintain a sense of optimism, reset a more appropriate task, do further groundwork in therapy and remain encouraging.

Sabotage by family members or friends is usually due to misunderstanding of the therapy. Particularly in patients with confirmed medical or suspected medical conditions, the family have often assumed a protective, caring role. They also often share in the patient's anxiety and may well feel nervous about some of the homework set, especially if it involves risk. They may also not have had the benefit of the rationale behind the homework. Sometimes, therefore, it is valuable to see key family members, with the patient, to clarify the issues and explain why the homework is safe and beneficial. This obviously can only take place with the patient's consent. This can also be helpful to get the precise plan for the homework across and family members can then provide encouragement. But it is important that encouragement and facilitation is all that is provided and that this does not develop into coercion or bullying. Some discussion with the family beforehand about how difficult the patient may find the task should prevent this.

Motivation can be a problem, particularly in patients who are depressed. Such patients may feel that however bad things are at present, at least they have got used to their situation. Trying something new, when they are generally pessimistic about the future, may seem fraught with problems, and they may well fear ending up in a worse place. It can also be very difficult to get started. Here the '5-minute rule' can be helpful. The patient is asked to try the task set for just 5 minutes; they can then choose to stop, but they should repeat the exercise on a regular basis. Of course, once 5 minutes is up they may well feel able to carry on for longer and make a real attempt at the task. On the other hand, they may quickly sink back into the same frame of mind, but they can use the same technique again, and gradually the task should become easier. Sometimes here it can be helpful to get them to assess their mood on a scale of 0 to 100 at various points in time – before they got started, at 5 minutes, and so on. This can also be done retrospectively, and when there is an improvement of mood on attempting the task, this can be linked back to the cognitive theory of emotion (see Chapter 2, p. 8).

As a conclusion, good homework helps the patient to take significant steps forward in therapy. It is important to construct appropriate tasks carefully and meaningfully with your patient. Take the time to get it right.

- Explain the reasons for homework carefully and get the patient to repeat what they have to do before they leave.
- Anticipate difficulties as much as possible by allowing different strategies to address the problems.
- Emphasise that homework is an important personal task and the therapist is privileged to see it.
- Reinforce successful homework strongly, even if at first it does not seem to be going well.
- Be prepared to be flexible if there are continued difficulties in getting the answers you need from successful homework.

Chapter messages

- Homework is essential with treatment, and should be introduced as the part of the treatment where the patient makes an original contribution by finding out new information and bringing it back to the therapist.
- Try to take into account all the barriers that might prevent homework being carried out and see whether you can anticipate them in setting the homework strategy.
- Always praise the patient for their homework efforts, no matter how small these are.
- If homework fails, blame yourself, not the patient, and try to modify it so it gets back on course.

CHAPTER 7

Setting goals

Goal-setting is an important way of marking progress for patients and instilling a sense of achievement. Goals elicit hope and when reached, demonstrate success.

Setting goals: short-term, medium-term, long-term

Goals can be short, medium and long term. They should be realistic, achievable and meaningful to the patient.

Short-term goals in the treatment of health anxiety can be related to the techniques used in therapy (e.g. being able to control excessive checking, or being able to resist looking up health issues on the internet; having successfully done the latter, a medium- or long-term goal could be using the internet again but being able to evaluate the information obtained in a non-threatening way).

Longer-term goals can be more difficult to set, as often patients with health anxiety cannot see a meaningful long-term future for themselves. They have just been preoccupied with illness or premature death. For this reason, it is important not to set these goals too early, that is to say, before the patient has started to make a cognitive shift. At the time the goals are made they should be seen as achievable, fitting in with the progress made in therapy.

Sometimes goals suggest themselves during therapy sessions. For example, the patient may say: 'Because of all my problems we've not been able to have a holiday for years. I feel bad about this because I know my wife would like to get away, if only to visit the children'. This particular comment immediately suggests two potential goals, a medium-term one to visit the children (which would probably seem a relatively safe start), and the possibility of a proper holiday on their own in the longer term. For this example, it may be too early to mention this as a goal, but it could be suggested: 'Has it been long since you visited? Would you like to be able to visit them again at some point?'. You could then note this down for bringing up at a later stage.

Some patients really struggle to come up with goals and often cannot produce one on the spot. You may have to provide suggestions, get them to talk about it with a relative or friend, or even ask that as we are all going to die one day, what would they like to be remembered for or what special thing would they like to have done. This approach may reveal some long-term goals that are only achievable well into the future after therapy has finished. A patient in one study whose long-term goal was to go travelling again was discovered to have done this when the GP notes were accessed a year later to collect the economic data in a research trial. Another patient with a similar goal was encouraged to send a postcard back to the therapist when he and his wife went on their holiday, which they duly did!

Problems encountered and resetting goals

It is obviously important that goals are achieved, so care must be taken when setting them with the patient. Together, check that the goal is the desired one, anticipate hurdles, discuss ways of overcoming them and set a realistic time frame. Remember to ask about how they got on because they will have invested a lot in this! When the goal is achieved remember to give them praise and ask them how difficult it was to manage, acknowledging the effort involved and the progress made, in other words 'flag it up'; it is a significant milestone in treatment.

If a goal has not been achieved, share the responsibility for that, discussing the setbacks, and accept that it may be you who got it wrong. It might have been your goal rather than the patient's, it might have been too taxing or the wrong time, or perhaps there were some unexpected obstacles. You may need to start again, so do not flog a dead horse!

Chapter messages

- Setting goals is important, as otherwise treatment can become unfocused.
- Always set goals collaboratively, do not impose them on the patient.
- Try to split goals into long-term and short-term ones.
- If it does not seem possible to set goals initially, then return to them again during therapy.

CHAPTER 8

Relapse prevention

Patients frequently experience a period of relapse, even if it is only short. Discussion around this possibility is a crucial part of therapy. It should be done before therapy sessions are concluded, as the patient still needs to feel that they have some support. This may be triggered by a new health scare of some kind or some other external pressure, such as stress at work. It can be opportune if this occurs within the period of therapy so that further work can be undertaken to cope with potential problems in the future. Sometimes the last therapy session can be set at a more distant time in the future to allow for this.

Breaking down the problem into sets of potential triggers, followed by early warning signs of these, can help your patient to start to put in place the new skills that they have learnt in therapy straight away, and they can learn from the experience. It is also important for them to realise when and how they can ask for help. If the problem seems overpowering they need to be able to contact you, their therapist, or perhaps their GP, who should be aware of the problem early on. But they can also take the step of contacting you to explain they are having difficulties, outlining what they are doing to cope, so at least they know you are aware of the problem. Remember to recognise that they are trying to work through it on their own, and encourage them to contact you when they have got through it so you can congratulate them on how they have done. It is helpful to emphasise that a relapse is not going to be as bad, or last as long, as the initial illness and that they are in a better place now with new skills and beliefs.

Identifying potential triggers for relapse

Although the details of these are highly specific to your patient, there are some general pointers for all patients. Any major life event, such as a promotion at work, loss of a job, financial pressures, relationship difficulties, illness in family or friends, or the increased responsibility of having a child can trigger a relapse (see Case example 8.1).

Case example 8.1: Health anxiety relating to pressures at work

Josh had a very successful business career; he was the technical trouble-shooter for a major company and very well thought of at work. He had developed health anxiety when a protégé of his died at work while he was on holiday. He was devastated on his return that he had not been there at the time, and felt very guilty that he had been on holiday enjoying himself while his young colleague lay dying. Josh developed terrible headaches and had a period off work, following which he requested a move to a different branch, which was granted. He was convinced he had developed a brain tumour and was a constant visitor at the doctor's, undergoing extensive investigations, including a brain scan, which was negative. He avoided going out with his friends or accompanying his wife on family gatherings, preferring to stay at home to avoid having to tell them he thought he was dying. One Christmas was particularly bad, as he had flu and he interpreted this as evidence of terminal illness.

Josh did well in therapy, but realised that many of his other worries were related to the possibility of promotion within the firm. He was very well regarded at work and tended to take on the jobs of others as he was so adept, and was frequently asked for advice. His manager was keen to reward him as he was doing a lot extra already without, in his opinion, sufficient financial reward. Promotion would, however, bring the extra responsibility of dealing with redundancies and firing staff who were not up to the job. Josh had made up his mind that he was going to resist this, but every 6 months when the subject came up he became very anxious and his worries about health worsened again. He also realised that other triggers were present, so that even a minor illness such as a cold made him feel vulnerable. In addition, he started to realise that any hint of bad news upset him too.

Recognition of these triggers was quite revealing and he started to feel that he understood himself a lot more; the worries began to seem less of a threat.

Recognising the early signs of relapse

This is an important skill, and again, highly personal. For Josh from Case example 8.1, these constituted re-emergence of the headaches, accompanied by other symptoms of anxiety such as dizziness and sweating. Difficulty getting off to sleep was another sign, as were trying to avoid social gatherings and feeling irritable.

Utilising the new skills from therapy to manage the relapse

Here patients are encouraged to look through the work they have done in therapy and repeat some of the exercises with respect to their current situation. In Josh's case, he found writing down his thoughts and emailing them to his home address helped him to address the problem early on. He also realised that telling his wife or his best mate at work that he was feeling under pressure, rather than bottling things up, helped him to feel supported, and things seemed less threatening. It also helped him to recognise that he could take time to work through a problem, especially if it was work-related; he did not have to come up with an instant solution.

When to ask for help

Deciding to seek help can pose a big problem for some patients. Contacting a health professional in times of difficulty could represent reassurance-seeking, which throughout this book we have shown is counterproductive in a number of ways. Expressing the difficulties the person is having is a different matter. The content of the fear may not need to be directly addressed. The patient can be asked to make sense of the fear themselves, using the techniques they have developed. This approach encourages the patient's developing autonomy, and although the therapist's involvement has to be flexible, mirroring the degree of distress, the process is designed to help the patient help themselves.

Josh understood that if his new-found techniques at work seemed really unsafe or that he was not able to concentrate and put them into practice, he should ask for support. He also realised that in the workplace he should ask for time or extra support in his routine work if there was a particularly demanding problem that had surfaced.

He also concluded that asking for help was not a last-ditch approach – it could be entirely sensible and reasonable, a conclusion he had never reached before. He also realised that there were many times when people valued being asked for help, and that in fact he was just practising what he preached.

Lessons to learn from the experience

The whole approach of CBT is learning to do things in a different, less threatening way, and the stress is on the word 'learning'. It takes time and practice to do things differently, and time to appreciate the benefits. An episode of relapse is not necessarily a bad thing; when worked through successfully, it can strengthen your patient's belief in themselves and their ability to overcome any future problems.

One of Josh's main conclusions here was that he did not need to see his anxieties as a sign of weakness; they could be interpreted as a sense of wanting to do the best he could, but that things had just gone a bit too far. He also realised that although the techniques were straightforward, it was important not to jump the gun, but to work through each worry properly in stages from the start. Time spent doing this was well worth it. He appreciated the importance of remembering just how much progress he had made, and how good he felt when the headache finally went and he realised that there was nothing medically wrong. There was a huge sense of liberation and he felt he must take care not to lose that.

Chapter messages

- Short relapses are very frequent in the treatment of health anxiety, and the patient should be advised to expect these.
- When relapses occur, try to identify the triggers that precipitate them.
- Use relapse positively and make it a learning process in which new information has been obtained that could be very helpful in the long run.
- Remember to emphasise the negative value of external reassurance when relapses occur and try to replace this with internal reassurance in which the patient takes control.

CHAPTER 9

Troubleshooting

Psychiatric comorbidity: depression, generalised anxiety, obsessive–compulsive disorder, bereavement, panic

The diagnosis of health anxiety overlaps with other anxiety disorders such as generalised anxiety and panic; patients may also have depression. This associated pathology may also need to be addressed with a cognitive–behavioural approach. Comorbidity with confirmed organic pathology is also common and not a barrier to CBT; the major consequence of comorbidity is likely to be a modification in the form of behavioural experiments, and clarification with those directly responsible for the medical care of these patients is necessary in most cases. Other comorbidities such as psychosis, substance misuse or eating disorders may complicate therapy, necessitating referral for more specialist care.

There may also be issues surrounding bereavement or relationship difficulties that need to be addressed, and sometimes, particularly in individuals with comorbid organic pathology, fears regarding employment.

Excessive rumination

Some patients spend an enormous amount of time going over and over their worries in their minds. They find it hard to concentrate on anything else and can feel exhausted and depressed as a result. This can be a difficult symptom to control, but it can be helpful to ask the patient to consider thinking about the problem in the most worrying terms, telling you about it for 5 minutes. You ask them to rate their mood at the beginning and after the 5 minutes, when it will inevitably be lower, linking it to the cognitive theory of emotion (see Chapter 2, p. 8). You then ask them to consider a less threatening scenario, which you help them to construct. You can measure mood again after this, although initially it can be hard to find the scenario convincing. As homework they are asked to work on alternative scenarios, writing them down as fully as possible, then considering the relative merits of the two different interpretations.

Sometimes patients struggle to find an alternative, less threatening sequence of events, in which case special attention in therapy should be given to this in order to overcome rumination.

Liaising with medical services

It is always important for the therapist to liaise with the patient's GP and the specialists in secondary care. Sometimes it is necessary to discuss the need for further tests and investigations, as often these are generated by patient pressure rather than clinical need and can itself compound the problem. In addition, advice to monitor a problem can become another problem in itself. An anxious patient who is advised to check his sputum all the time can become obsessed by this, examining it minutely many times a day and often inducing expectoration as a form of reassurance-seeking. Far from being helpful, this kind of advice tends to make the problem worse by focusing the patient's attention on possible ill health all the time.

Dealing with family and friends

Patients with health anxiety rarely keep their fears to themselves, although they may try to minimise the effect, particularly on their children. They may transmit the fears to other family members, but more often they involve them in reassurance-seeking. Health-anxious patients, unless they are avoidant, regularly seek medical advice from professionals, and although this often provides relief it tends to be only very short lived. Reassurance can almost prove addictive, and so people also tend to seek reassurance from all those around them, and this becomes part of the problem. Families often unwittingly collude with these demands as they are only too willing to reassure their loved one that there is nothing wrong. However, the need for this attention can become incessant and difficult for others to cope with.

For example, patients who fear skin cancer often notice every tiny mark on their body, may ask their partners to check them too, all the time, and may constantly ask if any one particular mark is getting bigger or not. This not only focuses more attention on the problem, but can carry a considerable burden for the partner, and they can start to feel worried and uncertain too. The continual preoccupation with health can lead to breakdown in relationships. A health-anxious partner, never able to properly relax and enjoy themselves, can become a very wearing companion.

It is important to recognise these issues in therapy, and it may be necessary to see family members too, with the permission of the patient. An explanation of how health-anxious patients tend to think and why they cannot just 'snap out of it' can be very valuable to a frustrated partner. Collusion over checking and giving reassurance also needs to be addressed with the family. A patient's partner can still be comforting and supportive, while saying they are helping by not reinforcing the checking behaviour.

Getting stuck in therapy

Your patient may be encountering other problems, which may hinder their health-anxiety therapy, such as feelings of guilt, difficult family relationships or difficulties at work. These issues should be addressed for the therapy to progress, either alongside health anxiety or as separate problems (Fig. 9.1 and Fig. 9.2).

Dealing with requests for further tests or investigations

Sometimes patients may ask the therapist if they can arrange or re-refer them for further tests. This may be because they have developed a new symptom or sensation, or heard about a new test for their particular condition, or simply because they believe having one more test would 'make them certain once and for all'. Such requests invariably fall under the heading of reassurance-seeking, which needs to be identified as such and discussed with the patient, and are invariably not medically justified. What is more, anxiety can be created by further tests. These can induce more worry in the patient, first anticipating and then waiting for the results, coupled with the uncertainty generated by the doctor colluding with the patient's need for further reassurance. This not only undermines your therapeutic interventions but will make the patient feel worse.

There may be occasional exceptions, for example having a follow-up HIV test outside the window period for a genuine risk, and there may be

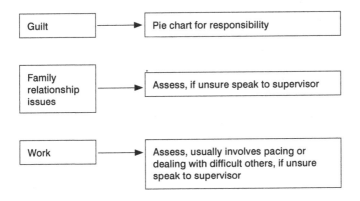

Fig. 9.1 Other issues emerging in therapy.

long-term monitoring of chronic conditions, but these have usually already been programmed into the care for that patient and as such are not requests for reassurance.

Some patients can appear to make a convincing case for re-testing or re-referral, in which case it is helpful to use the model outlined in Box 9.1,

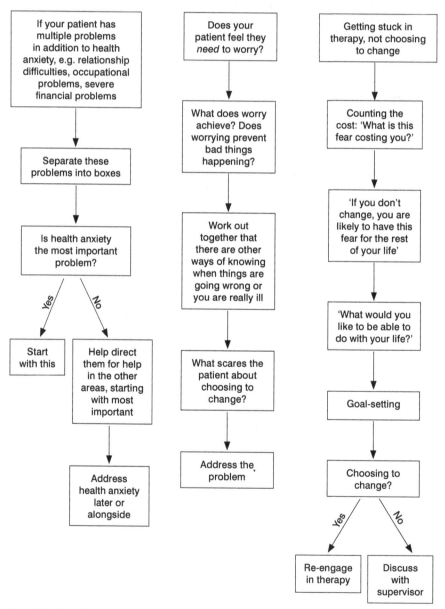

Fig. 9.2 Troubleshooting for various problems.

explaining why you are doing this with the patient. This model tends to go down well with patients. For one thing, it shows that you are considering their complaint on medical grounds and not dismissing it out of hand, but above all, you are helping them feel safe and understood without blanket reassurance. You are also helping them indirectly by illustrating how to weigh up symptoms and balance risk.

Box 9.1   Aid to testing relevance of symptoms to disease

You ask the patient to imagine that they have an identical twin, identical in every way, with exactly the same symptoms and sensations as your patient *except* that they do not worry about their health. You then explain that you are going to consider whether this identical twin, with the same symptoms, in the absence of anxiety, requires further testing. If you as the therapist feel that they do, then you will proceed with further investigations. If not, then you will defer; in this way you are weighing up the merits of further tests on medical grounds alone as opposed to only retesting because you are driven by your patient's anxiety.

Chapter messages

- Health anxiety is often associated with other physical and mental health problems.
- These problems may influence health anxiety and cannot be ignored, but may need to be treated differently from the anxiety.
- Repeated reassurance-seeking can undermine progress and may need to be managed in different ways, but do this by agreement with the patient, not unilaterally.

Part II

Presentation and aspects of management of health anxiety, by medical specialty

This section deals in more depth with problems more specific to certain areas of medicine, using case examples to highlight particular difficulties. However, the underlying principles of therapy are the same for each of these areas.

CHAPTER 10

Cardiology

Palpitations

Most patients attending cardiology clinics will complain of, or experience, palpitations. This may be their sole presentation or coexist with other symptoms. Palpitations are the conscious awareness of the heart beating. They can vary in speed and rhythm, can be regular or irregular, and tend to be episodic.

Palpitations occur naturally on exercise and in situations that induce a high state of arousal, such as fear or excitement; they can also occur with a fever. Palpitations can also be associated with alcohol withdrawal or a consequence of taking large amounts of caffeine, classically in strong tea or coffee. In some individuals they can also give the sensation of an occasional missed heartbeat due to harmless, naturally occurring, benign extra beats (extrasystoles), where a delayed heart beat is compensated for by a stronger one following; these can also be accentuated by stimulants such as caffeine.

Palpitations can be natural, normal phenomena, but of course may also be present at times in people with confirmed heart disease; most clinically significant palpitations are associated with ischaemic heart disease, thyroid disease and valvular heart disease.

But, and this is a very big 'but', they are also *very* common in anxiety.

Clinically significant causes of palpitations include:

- sinus tachycardia (fast regular heart rate due to conditions such as anaemia, heart failure, thyroid disease, infection);
- atrial fibrillation (very common, especially in the elderly, often in the presence of ischaemic heart disease; diagnosed by an electrocardiogram (ECG), but may be intermittent and so only detected on 24-hour recordings; patients may need anticoagulants to avoid strokes);
- Wolff–Parkinson–White syndrome (a form of rapid heart rate also diagnosed by ECG and usually harmless, although occasionally it is troublesome and may require surgical intervention);
- paroxysmal atrial tachycardia (can occur in all ages and is usually harmless; much more serious is ventricular tachycardia – it can require surgery and/or a pacemaker);

- ectopic beats (these are similar to benign extrasystoles, but here the underlying cause is ischaemic heart disease or thyrotoxicosis);
- heart block (conduction abnormality causing a very slow heart rate, may require a pacemaker);
- other rarer arrhythmias.

Almost all patients attending cardiac out-patient clinics complain of palpitations. They will all have received an ECG and been clinically assessed for the medical conditions described above, backed up by blood tests and in some instances with ultrasound tests or 24-hour ECG recordings. They may have had more invasive investigations such as angiography performed. Many of these patients will be diagnosed with medically unexplained palpitations (although this is not a formal diagnosis), and some of them will have high health anxiety and no serious pathology. Basically, the palpitations are a different form of the expression of anxiety, but one that is suspected to be a primary medical experience, and so when anxiety is mentioned, it is assumed to be a consequence of the palpitations, not the cause (Tyrer, 1973). It is also very important to know that patients can have underlying heart disease such as ischaemic heart disease, yet have palpitations that are entirely unrelated to this and so are benign.

We can then divide patients into two groups, those in whom the palpitations are caused by significant pathology or have another clear explanation (e.g. Wolff–Parkinson–White syndrome) and those in whom no cause is found. For some of these patients an underlying cause may be suspected, particularly if the symptoms are intermittent, but have failed to show on repeated 24-hour ECG recordings, but most patients have been given the medical 'all-clear' and told that the palpitations are 'nothing serious'. For both groups, where no clear cause has been found the most likely explanation is anxiety, but often this has not been explained in any meaningful way. For a person without health anxiety the reassurance is usually sufficient and their symptoms may gradually settle or stop causing concern. It is quite a different matter for those who worry about their health. In the absence of a clear explanation, they suspect there must be an underlying problem that the doctor has missed. Even in those patients for whom the diagnosis of some form of anxiety has been raised, individuals with health anxiety are likely to remain sceptical, particularly if the palpitations are a relatively new phenomenon that is out of keeping with their previous experiences.

In addition, patients who have underlying heart disease may notice more marked palpitations at times of stress, where the exacerbation of symptoms may be brought about by the higher levels of anxiety, and not, as is often suspected, evidence of new heart disease.

Evaluating and interpreting symptoms

For health-anxious patients, palpitations can be unpleasant and alarming, and the patient may find it difficult to accept them as normal or non-threatening. When they occur they tend to generate fears, such as 'my heart must be under strain' or 'I might be about to have a heart attack'. Such thoughts are clearly very frightening and so raise anxiety levels further, both perpetuating and reinforcing the palpitations. Extrasystoles, in addition, tend to create the sensation that the heart might be about to stop. These sensations drive the desire to monitor the heart rate or to check that the heart is still beating, usually by feeling the pulse or by placing a hand on the chest wall, over the heart.

There are also health anxious patients who learn to 'listen in' to their heart, managing to tune into their heart rate without checking their pulse (Case example 10.1).

Case example 10.1: A man with an irregular heartbeat

Mark was a 19-year-old student who over the past 3 years had become increasingly worried about his heart. A lot of the time he was conscious of it beating and occasionally noticed irregular beats. He was very fit and spent a lot of time in the gym or training on the running track, where he intensively monitored his breathing and listened in to his heart. He compared himself to others in terms of fitness and if he felt he was performing less well, became very anxious that his heart was not working hard enough. Paradoxically, he also worried that his heart never stopped to have a rest, and he wondered at times how on earth it kept going. If he noticed an irregular beat he became intensely anxious, thinking this was a sign that his heart now needed to stop. Occasionally, he got really angry about his heart and his preoccupation with it and went out running wearing three coats and heavy boots to really put it to the test.

Mark had also started to worry about the 'sudden adult death syndrome' and became preoccupied with media reports about footballers who had collapsed and died on the pitch where there had been no prior knowledge of heart disease, looking up further coverage of these stories on the internet. At one stage during the interview he performed a graphic demonstration of how one particular footballer had died.

He was becoming increasingly anxious and distressed by how this monitoring was dominating his life, but no matter how much be tried to push the fears away, they always immediately returned.

Clarifying past medical communications

The general public are now increasingly being encouraged to present early with symptoms that could relate to heart disease or stroke, so these patients feel it is imperative to act, even if they have been told in the past there was nothing wrong, just in case *this time* some pathology will be found.

Sometimes minor abnormalities are found on blood tests or ECGs, and if the patient is initially seen by a relatively junior doctor in emergency care, the tendency will be to treat the patient as if they have had a genuine cardiac event, which generates further anxiety. The patient may subsequently be told that everything is OK, but the process sends out a very mixed message and does not explain the symptoms.

Under these circumstances it is important to clarify the position with the consultant responsible for the patient that the symptoms are indeed completely, or at least partially, medically unexplained, so that the alternative hypothesis – that anxiety is contributing to the problem – can be explored.

Where there is underlying pathology, clarification is required about what the patient can be realistically expected to achieve, especially in terms of exercise tolerance.

Developing a formulation

Once the physician has excluded significant underlying pathology to account for their palpitations, careful evaluation of the patient's experience of previous episodes of these is paramount. A particularly severe episode of palpitations can be used to develop a formulation; this allows for the opening up of discussion regarding the beliefs and fears of the patient, starting to make sense of what these experiences mean for them. This often exposes misunderstandings which can be discussed, leading to basic education on the nature of palpitations, as described earlier. See Case example 10.2.

Case example 10.2: A woman with palpitations

Barbara, a 52-year-old secretary, had had health problems ever since she was a child. She could remember lying in bed at night listening to her heart beating, checking it would keep going while she was asleep so that she would still be alive in the morning. This had developed, when a teenager, into occasional episodes of irregular palpitations, which had persisted throughout Barbara's life, causing her concern.

Things had not been helped by being diagnosed as a child with a blood-clotting disorder, which had necessitated a series of blood transfusions over the years. Barbara had experienced numerous other fears about her health over the years, but these had escalated tremendously over the previous 18 months, after she had been diagnosed with mild coronary heart disease.

The problem began when, during a routine blood test for her blood disorder, Barbara casually mentioned to her GP that she had been a bit breathless at the swimming baths. She became very alarmed when the GP suggested that she should see a cardiologist. Almost immediately after her appointment with the GP her palpitations became more pronounced, adding to the concerns she had over her heart. Although she performed reasonably well during the treadmill test organised by the consultant, towards the end the tracing did show some ECG changes consistent with a degree of angina. A subsequent angiogram revealed a mild degree of coronary artery disease, but because intervention in the form of surgery was contraindicated by her blood disorder, she was managed on medication.

Following this diagnosis she was consumed with anxiety. Her irregular palpitations, diagnosed as benign extrasystoles by the consultant, became much more troublesome, dominating her life, and on occasions leading to emergency admissions to hospital, where she was monitored overnight and then discharged.

During development of the formulation for a particularly distressing episode of palpitations, at the beginning of her CBT therapy, she revealed that she believed the palpitations indicated that her heart was undergoing great strain and that she might die of a heart attack at any moment. These thoughts were coloured by images of herself gasping for breath, knowing that she was going to die, very shortly leaving her husband to cope alone for the rest of his life. Activities such as preoccupation with listening to her heart and checking her pulse to make sure it was still beating, were also readily identified in the formulation.

Employing CBT techniques

In my work, I often find that recording a diary of when the palpitations occur, what the patient was doing when they occurred and what the sensation meant for them at the time provides the basis for linking the symptoms to distress or anxiety. An example of how to do this can be based on a detailed retrospective account of a previous episode (e.g. 'Tell me what happened first. What were you doing at the time? What went through your mind when you noticed your heart beating? What did the fear do to the sensations?', and so on). The account gained in this way is followed up by the diary given as homework, which can help when patients struggle to remember things clearly. The diary should also include recording daily activities alongside the episodes of palpitations, and what the patient does to manage it at the time; for example, do they monitor their heart rate, do they go and lie down, and so on? Patients are also asked to record their thoughts during these episodes. Initially, many are unable to do this, in which case they are asked to record their thoughts immediately afterwards; what did they think was causing the sensations, what did they feel they should do, how safe or unsafe did they feel? They may have developed recurrent patterns of behaviour involving other worried family members, such as asking a family member to observe them or check their pulse, and if possible, this should be recorded too.

Careful examination of a diary of the palpitations and a history of previous attacks can allow the symptom to be built into the formulation, if not already there. It can be helpful to develop a formulation based on a particularly severe or frightening bout of palpitations. This should identify triggers such as upsetting thoughts or drinking caffeine-containing drinks (patterns from the diary can be particularly helpful here). It should also illustrate safety-seeking behaviours developed by the patient, for example, lying down until the palpitations have passed. These reinforce the illness model and the idea that rest is helpful, preventing anything worse happening.

Looking through the diary and examining the formulation in this way can lead into discussion of the part fear has to play in the development and maintenance of the palpitations. It can be helpful to ask the patient to complete the Beck Anxiety Inventory (a good standard measure of recording anxiety; see Chapter 5, pp. 52–53) for an episode of palpitations, allowing them to identify how many other symptoms of anxiety are present at the time, building the case for the anxiety model.

The problems associated with palpitations often interfere significantly with a patient's life, and although they tend to be, on the whole, slightly less problematic or dramatic than episodes of non-cardiac chest pain, the exercise of considering the cost of having a life dominated by these episodes can be a useful one.

Behavioural experiments

The patient is then invited to test out the evidence for the anxiety model by looking at the effects that checking and other safety-seeking behaviours have on focusing attention on the problem and hence tending to maintain it. For example, they could monitor their pulse regularly (and especially during attacks) while recording their anxiety through the day for 2 days, and then see what happened to their anxiety on days when they did not check at all.

If it looks as if there might be an association between episodes of palpitations and the ingestion of caffeine, the patient could carry out an experiment of recording palpitations on days when they drank a lot of coffee and on days when they cut out caffeine and other stimulants completely.

Here we can pick up again on the example of Barbara (Case example 10.2, continued).

Case example 10.2, continued

Barbara was asked to complete a diary for these events and what she was doing at the time they were experienced. This revealed over the course of a week that her palpitations were particularly troublesome at times of stress. Further examination of the diary also indicated that the palpitations tended to occur at times when she was at a loose end as well as at times of anxiety, and they did not occur when she was occupied and busy at work. It was also noted that there was probably a relationship to drinking coffee.

She was thus invited to consider whether she was experiencing the 'fear of having a heart attack' during these episodes as opposed to actually having heart problems, and to consider the evidence for this. Discussion around the effects of checking led to increased checking of her pulse for 2 consecutive days, followed by cessation of checking for the rest of the week while she monitored her anxiety. There was some reduction of anxiety on the days when she resisted checking, but not as much as might have been expected. However, this was readily explained by the fact that she was still able to monitor her heart by her learnt technique of listening to it, which she had perfected as a child.

Linking up episodes of severe palpitations to times of particular stress revealed that the palpitations had been worst of all during her angiogram. Interestingly, during this serious, complex, invasive investigation, a cardiac monitor is always constantly recording and is scrutinised by the senior clinician performing the procedure, so that any problem with the ECG would be immediately noted and acted on. She verified that this had indeed occurred, and even mentioned that she could identify her extra heartbeats on the screen. This led to the following conversation:

Therapist: So your heart rate was being constantly monitored throughout the procedure?
Patient: Yes, they were watching it all the time, alongside the picture of my heart and where the catheter was going.
Therapist: Could you identify the extra heartbeats on the screen?
Patient: Oh yes, it was terrifying, I thought my heart was going to stop any moment!

Therapist: Would the doctor have seen these too?

Patient: Yes, you couldn't miss them!

Therapist: Did he comment on them?

Patient: No.

Therapist: So you were having these extra beats on the screen during this invasive procedure, and a procedure not without risk, and the doctor didn't mention them. How concerned then do you think he was about these irregular beats?

Patient: Well… I suppose he wasn't all that concerned, actually he seemed quite relaxed, he even chatted to me at times.

Therapist: So do you think he feels they are a cause for concern?

Patient: Well no; I suppose I'd never thought about it like that before.

She was then asked to complete the Beck Anxiety Inventory for an episode of severe palpitations to see whether any other features of anxiety were present at the same time (many were), again building up the case for fear of disease.

Further homework was set, asking Barbara to find other evidence from things in the past to support the theory that these palpitations were in fact a benign phenomenon, as the consultant had explained, and thus normal for her, supporting the 'fear of disease' model. She was also encouraged to resist checking and specifically to resist 'listening in' to her heart.

She returned a week later with a long list of reasons why the palpitations were normal for her, including the fact that they had been there all her life, and that she had never had anything serious happen as a result. She also noted that they went away on their own. Not surprisingly, she also reported that they had settled down a lot, in fact only occurring once in the week, and then only briefly, after an espresso coffee during a meal out.

Common problems encountered in management

Sometimes family members and friends have developed an overprotective role with health-anxious patients, encouraging them to rest and avoid any activity or stress that could precipitate an attack. In those patients in whom a bout of palpitations might indicate an imminent stroke or a heart attack, involvement of other agencies and/or relatives, with the patient's agreement, may be useful.

There may be an association with breathlessness (see Chapter 11) and non-cardiac chest pain, and these should be addressed alongside the palpitations.

Chest pain

Chest pain indicating a heart attack is typically described as central, crushing and radiating into the left arm or the jaw, and is often accompanied by pallor and sweating. This type of presentation is by no means universal, and sometimes a myocardial infarction (commonly known as a heart attack) can be silent, in that it produces no obvious symptoms. Huge publicity campaigns stress the importance of early recognition of a potential myocardial infarction, as swift medical intervention greatly reduces morbidity and mortality.

Emergency departments have standard immediate procedures to diagnose and treat a myocardial infarction, and once the diagnosis is suspected, the patient is treated for a myocardial infarction before the confirmatory results (usually in the form of blood tests for raised cardiac enzymes) are received. Patients in whom ECG changes are apparent may also receive emergency angiography, an invasive procedure where a catheter is introduced through a blood vessel in the leg into the coronary arteries and dye is injected to detect the degree of occlusion of the vessels, and to see whether any blood clot that may be forming can be dissolved before total loss of blood supply to the heart muscle occurs. The treatments are dramatic, well-rehearsed and life-saving in many situations. This approach is entirely reasonable, but where problems occur is when health-anxious patients attend with non-cardiac chest pain.

For patients with non-cardiac chest pain who present to emergency departments, the treatment, or more specifically the investigation, will at least initially be the same, and is often terrifying. They will be initially seen by more junior medical staff who, as a precaution, even if the patient had presented with what has been diagnosed as non-cardiac chest pain previously, will err on the side of caution and initiate the standard myocardial infarction pathway of care. Even if all tests are negative the patient is likely to have to stay in hospital (currently, for about 12 hours) while a troponin test is carried out. All these procedures tend to reinforce the patients' belief that they had been right to attend, and that even if nothing abnormal was found on that particular occasion, the next time it happened there most certainly would be. Patients are often encouraged to present to the emergency department again if they experience chest pain, often saying 'in case the next time the pain is due to your heart'. Non-cardiac chest pain is also common in those who have proven existing heart disease. They may have had previously diagnosed angina or even a myocardial infarction, and have had treatment in the form of stents to keep the damaged arteries patent, or they may have undergone coronary artery bypass surgery. However, the whole experience may have proved very traumatic and for some who develop health anxiety, far from feeling 'treated successfully', they may become terrified of experiencing another cardiac episode, monitoring their body all the time for any evidence to support this and seeking help at the earliest opportunity.

Clarifying past medical communications

For many patients who have been given the all-clear after an episode of chest pain, the initial sense of reassurance they receive soon wears off. They may feel puzzled by the lack of a clear explanation for what *did* cause the pain, or they may have been told it was due to panic or stress and advised to relax, which in the absence of a clear explanation of the fear is difficult to achieve. They will almost certainly have also been told to come back if they were to experience any chest pain in the future, giving very mixed messages to an already worried person.

Some patients who have had cardiac pathology and interventions for this attend courses for rehabilitation, which may include graded exercise programmes and relaxation exercises. These may be helpful for many patients, but they do not usually include individual exploration of patients' fears.

Patients are often told they can go back to living a 'normal life', but they may be fearful of this, feeling a lack of confidence around issues such as going back to work or resuming sexual intercourse, or perhaps even seemingly straightforward activities such as driving the car on their own. Avoiding such activities to be on the safe side can lead to a very restricted existence, of which the medical team may be completely unaware (see Case example 10.3).

Case example 10.3: Fear of a heart attack

Bernard, a man in his 60s who had recently taken early retirement, had been admitted to hospital with chest pain 10 months previously. He was told he had probably had 'a small heart attack' and underwent angiography a few weeks later to further assess the extent of his coronary artery disease. A single vessel was found to be partly blocked and he was fitted with a stent. He made a good recovery, was discharged home and told to live a normal life.

Bernard had previously been fit and well, a non-smoker, and enjoyed walking, gardening and looking after his chickens, which he kept in a coop at the bottom of his long garden. Once a week he also liked to go to the social club with his son-in-law and play pool. The only additional advice he had been given was to try to lose weight, and he had been started on medication for mildly raised serum lipids.

After returning home, Bernard felt dreadful. He had never imagined he would develop heart disease and the whole experience in hospital had terrified him. He felt he now had to protect his heart so that it could not happen again, but in addition felt that he could be struck down at any time, like he had been before, and that this time help might not be immediately available. He gave up all his previous activities and took up a mostly sedentary life, confined to the house. His wife had taken some time off work when he was first discharged from hospital, but when she returned to work he began to experience panic attacks when she was out of the house, and rang her at her desk begging her to return. Eventually, his wife had to give up her job and remained at home with him, which led to a marked reduction in income. Bernard only really felt safe when he was in the house close to the telephone with his wife nearby. He felt the exertion of digging the garden was far too risky and his wife had to take over its maintenance; she also had to care for the chickens as the coop was a long way down the garden. Eventually, he became completely housebound and agoraphobic. His wife was also prevented by him from going out, unless someone he trusted could stay in the house with him. She was beginning to feel very isolated and depressed.

The only time Bernard left the house was to attend his 6-month follow-up appointment at the hospital. The medical team were pleased with the results of an exercise test and he was given a clean bill of health. They did advise him again to lose weight, but his lipids were now within the normal range and he was discharged back to the care of his GP. He had felt too embarrassed to disclose his fears or to ask any questions and the staff at the hospital had no idea how handicapped he had become. On returning home he was very upset that he had been discharged from the cardiology department, as this made him feel even more alone with his problem. He had rarely seen his GP, reinforcing the fear that he himself was the only person left to look after his heart now.

Evaluating and interpreting symptoms

Once a diagnosis of non-cardiac chest pain is made, clarification of what this means for the individual patient should be undertaken. Some patients may still believe that there is an underlying problem with their heart which requires further investigation, especially in the absence of any other explanation for the pain. They are usually reluctant, at least at first, to accept that anxiety could be contributing to the problem. Discussion with the consultant involved in their care and examination of the medical notes are important, especially as any psychological treatment may involve the patient exercising more.

Developing a formulation

Taking the patient back to a recent episode of pain and reliving the experience and what it meant for them is a useful building block for treatment (see Chapter 4, pp. 28–32 and Fig. 4.1).

Case example 10.4: Chest pain in someone who had previous heart disease

Marcus was a 58-year-old marketing consultant. He had always maintained his health reasonably well and had little cause for concern. Driving home from work one day, he began to feel unwell and a bit dizzy, and felt some tightness in his chest. He pulled off the road and telephoned his wife to say he felt very ill and could she call an ambulance. As he pulled in to the drive, he could hear the siren of the ambulance approaching, and as he walked into the house he collapsed on the kitchen floor. The next thing he was aware of was arriving in the accident and emergency department, where he was informed that he had had a heart attack and had been successfully resuscitated from a cardiac arrest. He made a good recovery and returned home, later undergoing successful angioplasty.

After his discharge Marcus began to experience frequent bouts of chest pain, necessitating readmission to hospital. On each occasion he was told that his heart was fine and he was discharged, but he had been unable to return to work. After several of these episodes he was referred for psychological evaluation and help.

A formulation for the most recent distressing episode revealed that in the late afternoon, while listening to the radio and hearing the news which he had always listened to in the car driving home from work, he began to feel dizzy and shaky. He immediately took his pulse and felt it was not very strong, and as he did this he experienced increasing tightness across his chest. He then became very frightened, thinking he was going to collapse, sat on a chair and phoned for an ambulance. He relived again the lucky escape he had had with his first heart attack, thinking that this time he would not be so lucky. While waiting for help he became increasingly certain that he was going to have another cardiac arrest and that he was going to die, before anyone could reach him, saying to himself, 'You couldn't be that lucky twice'. He was paralysed with fear.

Employing CBT techniques

For Marcus, his main fear was that he had been unbelievably lucky to have survived his cardiac arrest and that he had no such guarantee for the future. He was asked to complete a Beck Anxiety Inventory for his most recent distressing event, and it was noted that he was experiencing virtually every symptom of anxiety. He was asked to consider, especially in the light of his reassuring investigations on readmission, whether anxiety could be the possible cause of his symptoms. He was then invited to consider the Beck equation (see Chapter 2, p. 9).

Each aspect of the equation was addressed in turn. From his point of view, Marcus thought that it was exceedingly likely that if you have had one cardiac arrest you will have another (great likelihood of illness), and that next time he would die because it was a miracle he had been saved the first time (perceived awfulness). In addition, he felt he simply could not cope with anything anymore, he had lost all self-respect and he would never get back to work (no ability to cope with illness). He also felt that no treatment would make any difference, as although he was on medication now, he was still experiencing symptoms all the time (external factors cannot help).

To start with, Marcus was asked to consider the evidence that he would in fact be likely to have another cardiac arrest. On that occasion it was his first presentation of heart disease; he probably experienced an arrhythmia as a direct result of his acute myocardial infarction, but this had been addressed now, he was on treatment and the doctors had seen no evidence of any arrhythmias subsequently. He agreed that perhaps this was less likely than he had believed. He was then asked to reconsider the circumstances of the initial episode. His resuscitation had not been entirely due to luck, in fact he had recognised that he was seriously unwell and expeditiously organised the correct help, which had saved his life. He had in fact coped remarkably well in a life-threatening situation. In addition, his disease had been treated; he was carefully monitored and put on preventative treatment.

Being able to see his problem from a new, less threatening perspective and recognising that many of his symptoms could be attributed to excessive anxiety, led to a marked reduction in fear and, not surprisingly, in symptoms. Further consideration of the helpfulness of safety-seeking behaviours such as checking his pulse were considered, and when he stopped these his anxiety was further reduced. After a few weeks Marcus was able to return to work and listen to the news on the way home without reminders of the past.

Behavioural experiments

Behavioural experiments involved with the cessation of checking have already been discussed. Particularly relevant to cardiology patients is the extent with which they feel able to return to a 'normal life'. In the example of Bernard, he was asked to consider whether all his precautions had in fact saved any adverse event. He acknowledged reluctantly that in fact he had been symptom-free during the whole 10 months since his heart attack, apart from occasional episodes of panic. He felt that he wanted to get back to normal activities and expressed a desire to go to the social club and play pool. This failed dismally, as on arrival he was consumed with panic and unable to get out of the car and had to return home. A formulation of this episode revealed the extent to which he felt unsafe and the humiliation he would feel if he collapsed in front of his friends. A more graded exposure to leaving his safety zone was needed. Initially, he was encouraged to walk as far as the garden gate with his wife while his daughter stood by the telephone and watched from the window. This was rehearsed several times and he began to relax, even on one occasion feeling able to engage his neighbour in conversation. With the increased confidence this gave him, he managed to progress to walking to the gate alone and then going for a walk without telling his wife. Eventually, he was able to get out and about as usual and resumed his trips to the social club. This had been achieved after a discussion which illustrated that when he was at the club he would be surrounded by friends and that help would be readily available if required. He also recognised that he would be one of the first people to help anyone else, and in fact had been in that position in the past, when one of his friends had experienced a bad asthma attack. He had been pleased to help and certainly had not thought any the less of the person concerned.

Patients with health anxiety who attend cardiology clinics have recently been shown to benefit from having their anxiety addressed more than any other patients in other clinics (Tyrer *et al*, 2013), and successful treatment is also associated with much greater cost savings (Tyrer *et al*, 2011b). Cardiac rehabilitation nurses may find CBT particularly helpful for the patients they treat.

Common problems encountered in management

Cardiac events, whether suspected or confirmed, are terrifying not only for patients but also for the families. They have often accompanied the patient to emergency rooms and witnessed the seriousness with which they are treated by the paramedics and assessment team. They will have also been asked to wait outside while the patient is being treated for a suspected heart attack, and they will have been urged to bring the person back should they experience any further problems. They may well become overprotective as a result, compounding the problem, so the rationale behind the CBT needs to be carefully explained to them also, so that they can support the patient.

CHAPTER 11

Respiratory medicine

Respiratory diseases that may cause breathlessness

Breathlessness, or its medical term 'dyspnoea', is the prime complaint in respiratory medicine and a common complaint in cardiology. In this chapter we are considering primarily those patients who have been seen within respiratory medicine clinics, as those with breathlessness due to heart failure or coronary artery disease will tend to be seen in cardiology clinics, but obviously overlap between the specialties and conditions occurs.

Breathlessness is also a very common symptom of anxiety. It is a particularly frightening sensation, especially if patients feel that they are suffocating, and it is very easily misinterpreted as indicating underlying disease. Also, the anxiety generated by breathlessness occurring as a result of underlying respiratory or cardiac pathology can stimulate more fear, resulting in increased breathlessness due to superimposed hyperventilation.

One of the most common conditions encountered in out-patients is chronic bronchitis and its more severe consequences, chronic obstructive pulmonary disease (COPD) and emphysema, both of which are complicated by frequent superimposed chest infections. Asthma is also common, with wheezing as the predominant problem, but in some individuals attacks can be acute and very severe (there are occasional cases of sudden death in young people from asthma, and highly publicised cases such as these are often a major source of concern for the health anxious). Bronchiectasis is another chronic condition, where permanent lung damage is due to prior infection and it is characterised by the production of copious amounts of sputum; secondary infection is common here too. Cystic fibrosis is increasingly seen, as affected children now often survive into adulthood.

Other more acute conditions such as pneumonia and pulmonary embolus are often causes for concern as they are relatively common and well publicised. For example, advice is given repeatedly on how to prevent blood clots forming in the legs when flying to avoid a deep vein thrombosis and possible embolic complications. There are also repeated public health alarms about conditions such as bird flu and epidemics of diseases in different parts of the world that lead to special recommendations about travel. Lung cancer is also increasingly common and featured in endless campaigns, and although it does not usually present with breathlessness alone, this may develop in those with chronic obstructive pulmonary disease because of the established link with smoking, making it a very common fear. Phrenic nerve paralysis is another cause of shortness of breath, as in this condition the diaphragm cannot move to help expand the chest fully during respiration. It can occur as a complication of chest surgery.

Media highlighting of particularly topical conditions such as tuberculosis and lung cancer, and in recent years, of pneumocystis carinii pneumonia (PCP) in HIV/AIDS and mesothelioma (the form of lung cancer related to previous exposure to asbestos, often decades before) have generated major concerns in many health-anxious individuals. Other fears over occupational diseases such as pneumoconiosis or silicosis feature in populations where coal mining has been the predominant source of employment, with everyone in the community knowing stories of colleagues who have suffered from this.

For all these conditions, major contributory factors are a long history of smoking and weight gain. Many patients have stopped smoking when diagnosed with respiratory or cardiac disease, or after a 'scare', but many continue to smoke, unable to give up, or feeling that the damage is already done and there is no point in stopping now. (This is not true, continued smoking further impairs respiratory function, increases the risk of progression of disease and continues to increase the risk of developing lung cancer.) Sometimes younger people with health anxiety and possibly very little in the way of symptoms, also adopt this nihilistic attitude towards smoking, feeling the harm has already been done. Interestingly, many of these patients will spontaneously give up smoking as their anxiety is treated and they begin to feel optimistic about the future.

Breathlessness is common as an anxiety-related phenomenon, especially in a panic attack. It can also be found in generalised anxiety and adding to a pre-existing respiratory condition. It is usually manifest as hyperventilation or rapid breathing at the top of the chest, with the patient holding themselves tense, bracing themselves for something catastrophic such as a heart attack, collapse or death. It may be accompanied by feelings of suffocation where the patient feels there is insufficient air/oxygen in the room, and they must open a window, or, when it happens at night, that they must sit up or get out of bed and stand by the window to get more air. Some patients end up sleeping permanently in a chair or on the settee downstairs as a result of this. They become too frightened to go upstairs to sleep, needing to be near the door.

Some medical conditions such as acute heart failure are characterised by increased breathlessness on lying flat, particularly in the night, leading to the affected individuals requiring several pillows. Another example is sleep apnoea, where airflow into the lungs is interrupted for regular brief intervals throughout the night. However, such conditions are usually readily diagnosed and respond well to medical intervention.

When breathlessness occurs as a consequence of anxiety, the rapid, shallow breathing causes a disproportionate loss of carbon dioxide from the blood – 'hypocapnoea' – which manifests itself as tingling (usually in the hands or around the lips), dizziness and feeling light-headed, and wobbliness in the legs. Naturally, these associated symptoms further drive the thought that something catastrophic is about to occur, feeding into the cognitive theory of emotion model (see Chapter 2, p. 8).

Clarifying past medical communications

Many patients in respiratory medicine have disproportionate (and hence at least partially medically unexplained) breathlessness. Often it is thought by the physician in charge to be due to hyperventilation and this may have been explained to the patient. A simple explanation of hyperventilation or advice on trying not to overbreathe rarely helps in isolation. The absence of an exploration of any psychological component, for what is a terrifying symptom, is almost universally insufficient to improve the breathing or the distress it causes. Further efforts to try to help alleviate symptoms for these patients often go down the unnecessary pathway of trying new inhalers, or steroids, or providing them with a nebuliser device or oxygen at home. Of course, there are some circumstances where these measures are definitely medically indicated, but there are many where they are not, and the consultant, GP and the district or specialist nurses may become embroiled in futile attempts to make the patient feel better, which may, completely unintentionally, end up making them even more scared, out of control and disempowered.

Once health anxiety has been identified it is important to establish with the physician concerned the extent to which the patient might expect to be compromised by their medical condition, and to liaise with the other agencies concerned to establish a consistent supportive approach. This may involve ringing specific members of the team or arranging to meet them to discuss your assessment and planned way forward, and copying all the agencies and the patient in on any correspondence. See Case example 11.1.

Case example 11.1: Respiratory disease becomes respiratory anxiety

Jeremy was a 58-year-old man who had had successful cardiac bypass surgery for coronary artery disease 2 years previously. Unfortunately, however, the surgery was complicated by paralysis of the left phrenic nerve, making it harder to take deep breaths, but on the whole Jeremy made a good recovery. Shortly afterwards he was readmitted to hospital with a minor bleed from a peptic ulcer, which settled on conservative treatment. While in hospital, he unfortunately developed hospital-acquired pneumonia; this was serious and required three courses of antibiotics before he started to improve. Following this, he remained extremely short of breath most of the time, despite a documented 'full recovery' from the infection, with a clear X-ray.

At times, when his breathing difficulties were particularly severe, he also experienced associated tightness in his chest, and as a consequence of this, he had numerous admissions over the following year. However, nothing significant was detected and his breathlessness was out of all proportion to the clinical findings. Concern was also expressed that he was receiving too much radiation from his repeated chest X-rays.

Prior to the events of the past 2 years, Jeremy had led a full and active life. In addition to a faultless work record he had been a football enthusiast, supporting the local youth team as a coach and still playing himself at times. He was now retired from work and had not been to a game more than a couple of times since he had become ill. His life was confined to the house with long periods alone as his wife was still working. He spent most of the day on the settee, where he also slept so that he could remain in an upright posture without disturbing his wife. Close to the settee were his nebuliser and home oxygen supplies that he used at intervals during the day (and night), with little benefit. He also had a supply of steroids that his GP had advised he could take as a short course if he felt he was getting worse; he was never sure whether to take them or not, but erred on the side of caution and took one 'now and then'.

The specialist nurse visited him twice a week, advising him to check his sputum regularly to detect any early colour changes that might indicate infection, and to call her immediately if he felt worse in case he needed urgent hospitalisation. As a consequence, he spent many anxious hours each week wondering whether to call her or not, wondering whether he was deteriorating, for although he often felt he would be better off in hospital, on the last two admissions, when they had been unable to find much wrong, he had ended up feeling a fraud.

He felt now that he contributed nothing of any value any more, particularly at home, and had become a constant burden on his long-suffering, exhausted wife.

Evaluating and interpreting symptoms

The first stage involves taking a careful, detailed history and developing the formulation. Special consideration of problems surrounding the management of cases where there is underlying pathology is important. Clarification of the situation from the notes and the consultant in charge of their care is imperative. In many cases there is lack of clarity over the complexities of the medical issues, and where this confusion inevitably has filtered through to the patient, getting the patient to report back what was and was not said, and how it was interpreted. This is enormously helpful in developing a clear understanding of the current situation. Asking, 'How did you feel when the doctor said "there is nothing more we can do to help"?', and how the person interpreted this, is often very valuable. For the physician it might mean that: 'We've treated the wheeze and we've explained that the patient is making things worse by hyperventilating, but why he remains so ill is a bit of a mystery as we can't find anything else wrong to account for it'. The patient has a completely different conclusion: 'I'm too far gone for anything else to work, I'm never going to get any better. In fact, I will just continue to deteriorate until I die. I'm untreatable'.

Developing a formulation

Jeremy was identified as having high health anxiety, and the initial formulation of a recent severe bout of breathlessness and chest pain identified many patterns of behaviour and associated fears, including graphic, distressing images of his older brother. He had been discovered dead at home by Jeremy a week after he had been discharged from hospital after a bout of chest pain. The post-mortem had shown that he had died of a heart attack. This event had occurred prior to the onset of Jeremy's problems, but now, despite the fact that he had been told his heart surgery had been successful, he was increasingly fearful that he would die too. The next step was to contact the specialist nurse (with Jeremy's permission) to discuss his case and the way in which the therapist planned to proceed. Interestingly, this was greeted with great relief by the nurse who felt alarmed by Jeremy's clinical condition, while recognising his anxiety, but with no idea on how to deal with him other than monitoring his clinical condition as closely as possible.

Employing CBT techniques

When the breathlessness seems to be present a lot of the time, a better idea of when it occurs and what might be contributing to it can be obtained by keeping a diary, recording the degree of breathlessness and what was going on at the time. This breaks things up, giving a clearer picture, identifying fluctuations in symptoms and linking them to events, and sometimes it may identify periods when there is little or no breathlessness. The diary can be specifically tailored to the individual patient based on a hunch; for example, are the worst breathing difficulties experienced when the patient is on their own for a long period, or when they are away from the safety of home? This makes it important to record these activities too.

With the identification of the factors feeding into the anxiety model derived from the formulation, and the information derived from the diary, the patient is invited to consider the 'fear of' versus 'actually having' a severe disease accounting for their shortness of breath.

Behavioural experiments

In Jeremy's case, examination of the diary showed that his breathlessness was less noticeable when he was engaged in another activity, such as when his grandson visited and when he was watching football on the television, but it was worse when he was on his own at home during the day. Paradoxically, he was more active and excited chatting to his grandson and would go outside and watch him kick a ball about on the lawn; they were both also extremely animated when they watched TV together. During these times Jeremy thought less about his illness and rarely used his oxygen cylinder, and he also reported feeling much less anxious. Gradually, we were able to build up the link that feeling anxious and vulnerable induced the increased shortness of breath. This weakened the case for him having heart disease, and when he realised that watching his favourite team on TV in the grip of excitement did not lead to angina or worsening of his breathing, he began to realise that it was his *fear* of heart disease that was the problem.

Jeremy then began to consider how he could occupy himself more in the day, when his wife was at work. He felt guilty about how much she had to do and decided to take on a few more tasks himself, such as preparing the vegetables for the evening meal. As his confidence grew, he realised he was using his oxygen much less, and we discussed the possibility of moving it to a corner of the room rather than having it by the settee as a permanent reminder of illness. He was nervous of trying this at first, wondering what would happen if he needed it and could not get up from the sofa. As a first step he decided it could be in the corner when his wife or his grandson were there. This he managed surprisingly easily and everybody found it easier as there was a lot more room.

Checking his sputum for colour change, which might indicate infection, was also found to occupy a lot of Jeremy's time. He had previously used this phenomenon to alert him to the fact that he might need to go into hospital, but scrutinising things in this way, worrying if the spit was a shade darker or not, caused him a great deal of anxiety and led to admissions 'just to be sure'. However, on many of these admissions he had been reassured that there was no evidence of infection and had been discharged shortly afterwards. He felt humiliated by this and felt that he was wasting everyone's time.

After discussion with the district nurse, who had previously, in desperation, advised him to check the sputum, we decided to conduct an experiment to see whether checking was indeed helpful. Jeremy was asked to rate his anxiety throughout the day while checking his sputum at every available opportunity. He was then requested not to check at all for the rest of the week, but to continue to record his levels of anxiety in the same way. We discussed that it was safe to try this, because if he did develop a chest infection there would be other ways of detecting it, as he would feel ill, cough more and might have a temperature. We also discussed that it might be difficult not to check as it had become something of a habit, so if he did find that he had forgotten and checked he should record this too. He duly did the experiment and found that he worried less when he did not check and in fact, as the week went on, he could not be bothered to fill out the form any more. What is more, he and the family felt a lot better that there were no little pots of sputum around.

As his anxiety reduced and his confidence grew, Jeremy started to make a few tentative goals, initially to help his wife by accompanying her when she did some shopping (without the oxygen), and then to go and watch his grandson play football in a match. Achieving these led to him having the confidence to sleep upstairs again with his wife.

Common problems encountered in management

Breathlessness is a frightening symptom, not just for patients but for their families too, especially if they have been supplied with home oxygen and an easy route to readmission. Families often feel a huge sense of responsibility to get help, so when these beliefs about illness are challenged they need to be brought alongside too. Part of the process in therapy often involves a shift towards the patient taking responsibility for himself. When this is achieved, not only does it empower the patient, but it can often provide relief for those caring for them.

Inhalers and other devices commonly used in respiratory disease can be bulky and obvious, and act as a constant reminder of the problems with breathing. It may be helpful to avoid leaving cues like this on display.

Another common misconception in patients with respiratory problems is the feeling that there is insufficient oxygen in the room and that they need to open a window to let more in, especially at times when their breathing seems worse. Sometimes this occurs at night if they wake up and panic. Using lifts, for the same reason, can leave patients feeling that they are trapped inside and there will not be enough air. For someone who does have a degree of underlying respiratory impairment and would struggle with several flights of stairs, the inability to use a lift can place severe restrictions on their lifestyle. In these circumstances you ask them to consider that if you started to do some exercises in the room, would you need to open the door? You could then explain that the body's demand for oxygen increases dramatically with exercise and you could use yourself or another person to demonstrate that the air supply is completely sufficient. You could also ask the patient to consider why you never hear of people suffocating in a lift, despite them often being full, and ask whether air supply would be something that was considered in lift design.

The patient is then encouraged to try to resist opening the window, perhaps initially when they exercise a little and then when they are anxious, to show that when the fear passes they are still fine and have not collapsed for lack of air. They could then try using a lift, initially accompanied and only for one floor, gradually increasing the use and monitoring what happens (which is 'nothing much'). Avoiding lifts and opening windows are examples of safety-seeking behaviours which only serve to maintain the cycle of fear in health anxiety.

CHAPTER 12

Gastroenterology

Gastroenterological conditions that may cause health anxiety

Gastroenterological complaints feature frequently in patients with health anxiety and can be magnified in patients with underlying confirmed pathology because of superimposed anxiety.

Diseases that feature particularly prominently in media coverage are often the focus of these fears (in recent years, bowel cancer), and the extra screening associated with this where there is a strong family history. There are clear guidelines for such screening and investigations, but exceptions occur, particularly where patients have persistent troublesome symptoms or where they are unduly worried. Thus, many anxious patients may undergo unpleasant and unnecessary investigations, which at times will yield inconclusive or unclear results, adding to their fears.

Diagnostic labels such as 'irritable bowel syndrome', 'unexplained vomiting syndrome' (Case example 12.2, p. 104) and 'nutcracker oesophagus' are often given to complaints that are heavily associated with anxiety and largely unexplained. Often, patients cling to these labels, but this usually offers little in the way of relief and they tend to live lives dominated by these symptoms, frequently believing there is more severe underlying pathology that the doctor has failed to find.

Inflammatory bowel disease, in the form of Crohn's disease and ulcerative colitis, can cause huge disruption to patients' lives, and the anxiety generated by pain, troublesome diarrhoea and rectal bleeding can not only be difficult to cope with, but can also exacerbate the problem.

Clarifying past medical communications

Clear criteria guide physicians in terms of symptoms and the level of investigations required to exclude certain conditions, for the symptoms experienced are often very non-specific, such as altered bowel habit, cramping stomach pains or nausea, symptoms universally experienced from time to time by everyone. However, some symptoms are particularly distressing, such as rectal bleeding, where a small amount of blood from, for example, a small anal fissure (an anal tear often caused by constipation) or a small haemorrhoid can look quite alarming when dispersed by the water in the lavatory pan. Because many of these symptoms are so non-specific, there are often posters in the GP surgery and elsewhere, or notices in media coverage of medical matters, alerting patients to be vigilant for signs of possible underlying illness (e.g. bowel cancer) and not to ignore persistent episodes of bleeding (Case example 12.1).

Case example 12.1: Health anxiety about bowel cancer

Alison was a young woman who had recently had a baby. During her pregnancy she had been constipated a lot of the time and had developed a particularly troublesome rectal fissure, causing frequent small bleeds when she went to the toilet. She had always been health-anxious since a classmate at school died after eating some poisonous berries and the headmaster of the school issued a severe warning on the matter.

Her new responsibilities as a mother, combined with the worry of two maternal aunts being diagnosed with breast cancer, had led to the terrible conviction that she now had bowel cancer. She had also developed bouts of abdominal pain and on feeling her abdomen, thought at times that she had felt a lump, or possibly an enlarged liver. She had also noticed lumps on the side of her mouth which the dentist had been uncertain about, mentioning the need for a biopsy if they persisted. Frequent visits to the GP had resulted in a gastroenterological referral, where the fissure was identified as the cause for the bleeding, no abdominal mass was identified, and apart from some routine blood tests no further investigations were considered appropriate.

Alison was initially reassured by this but when one of the blood tests revealed a mild degree of iron deficiency anaemia, attributed to her recent pregnancy, all her fears returned with a vengeance. The iron tablets she was prescribed caused her to develop black stools and she became more constipated again, aggravating the fissure and exacerbating the episodes of bleeding. She was now visiting the toilet at every opportunity, examining the paper to assess the extent of any bleeding, and as soon as the baby went to sleep she logged on to the internet, desperate to find some reassurance, but ended up more convinced there was something seriously wrong. She also noticed that she was developing new symptoms, including nausea and headache, which to her suggested the disease was spreading and she might be developing secondary cancer.

She repeatedly visited the GP who attempted to reassure her, but in the course of this concluded that although she was not worried about Alison's bowels, she felt that, in view of the family history of breast cancer, Alison should be screened for this and possibly see a genetic counsellor. Alison left the consultation paralysed with fear, convinced that she was riddled with cancer from head to toe, spending hours in the toilet and checking her mouth and her skin, looking for, and often finding, marks that to her were suggestive of secondary deposits. The only thing she did not check was her breasts, which she had been specifically advised to examine on a monthly basis. She was simply far too terrified to do this, as she now felt almost certain a lump would be there.

Gastroenterological problems tend not to lead to as many emergency admissions as acute breathlessness or chest pain, but there are times when bouts of unexplained abdominal pain can be very severe, occasionally leading to admission and use of strong analgesics such as morphine, generating the expectation that this might need to be repeated with a subsequent admission. Compounding the problem is the fact that a clear diagnosis cannot really be made in medical terms, so the patient ends up receiving morphine under dramatic circumstances at one minute and then being discharged the next, having been told 'everything is normal' or even more misleadingly that there is 'nothing wrong'.

Evaluating and interpreting symptoms

A careful history is crucial to discovering the pattern and development of symptoms and to list the investigations and findings, identifying any ambiguities that may have arisen. Establishing patterns of symptom fluctuation over time can also be helpful, noting any associations with stressful life events. It is also important to ask about any specific dietary restrictions that patients may have imposed on themselves. These can be quite excessive at times, leaving the person unable to enjoy going out for a meal. Some patients are severely limited in the extent to which they can go out at all, for fear of having diarrhoea and being incontinent. This is true for irritable bowel syndrome and, of course, for all inflammatory bowel disease.

To assess all the components of these, and how they link into the symptoms, a diary is very useful. Again it is important to consider what information you want to obtain and tailor the diary accordingly.

Case example 12.2: Unexplained vomiting

Jennifer had been experiencing health anxiety for 3 years. It started soon after her teenage son began having problems at school; he was being bullied and had refused to attend for long periods. He also had asthma, which had been exacerbated by all the worry at school, and on one occasion had had to go to an emergency department to receive treatment for an acute attack. Jennifer had started developing quite severe epigastric pain associated with nausea and vomiting. Over the first 2 years she had had two endoscopies which were normal and had also had investigations for coeliac disease, but these were also clear. She was eventually diagnosed with 'unexplained vomiting syndrome', put on increasingly large doses of medication, including an anti-emetic cyclizine, which she was taking in larger doses than advised, and was experiencing troublesome side-effects (or withdrawal symptoms) of trembling. She had nausea every day and frequent bouts of vomiting bile; she could only go out if she had had nothing to eat on that day. Her symptoms had got worse in the past 6 months following a holiday abroad, where the illness had been particularly bad, although not thought to be due to any form of food poisoning. She had lost weight and over the previous 6 months had also developed an annoying hacking cough which had not responded to antibiotics. Her firm belief was that she had cancer with secondary deposits in her lungs.

A careful history revealed that the holiday had been particularly upsetting as it was the last holiday she and her husband had before they split up, and they had argued all the time. This information had been divulged during construction of the formulation. At this time the therapist observed that the holiday had also coincided with the worsening symptoms; Jennifer was quite surprised and agreed that she had been very stressed at the time.

She was due to receive further investigations shortly in the form of pressure studies on her oesophagus. This necessitated prior cessation of her medication, which terrified her as the vomiting was 'bound' to get worse.

Feelings of guilt are often found in association with inflammatory bowel disease, where patients frequently feel that they are being punished. One young Asian lady felt that she had developed ulcerative colitis as a punishment from the prophet Mohammed for having a termination of pregnancy. Another lady, Clare, felt that that her Crohn's disease had developed as punishment because of what she considered to be a terrible misdemeanour as a child. When aged about 10, she and a friend had stolen into an old churchyard and while playing there had picked dandelions and distributed them on all the graves. On the way home she wondered whether they should have done this, so she told her mother when she arrived back. Her mother was very angry indeed, saying that she had no business to go playing in such places as she was disturbing the dead, and she was sent to her room and forbidden to go to her friend's birthday party. She still found it incredibly difficult to talk about this event and remained mortified by what she had done. Her therapist explored other interpretations with her, and together they came to the conclusion that it was in fact a lovely thing to distribute the flowers, and any visitors to the graveyard would have been very touched by what they saw. In fact, the conclusion they both came to was that the whole event had been completely innocent and that she had been unfairly punished for it. This simple revelation, 19 years later, produced an almost overnight reduction in her symptoms. She experienced less abdominal cramps and an anal fistula (a long-standing complication of the disease) at last began to heal. She had an enormous gain in confidence, and also realised that young people developing inflammatory bowel disease could not possibly be blamed for their illness.

Developing a formulation

The formulation for Jennifer was centred around the day of the parents' evening at her son's school. She had woken up with this event as her first thought and had immediately begun to feel sick; she went downstairs and had half a piece of toast and a cup of tea, but then realised that she must not eat anything all day, otherwise she would be too ill to attend. She then thought about how much her life was constrained by her problems and felt guilty about neglecting her son, never having much fun with him, and guilty over the break-up of her marriage. She 'knew' that she was getting worse and felt her throat and her stomach to check for lumps and tenderness. When she pressed her stomach, she felt sick again. On going to the bathroom, after retching in the sink, she looked in the mirror and felt she had lost even more weight and that she was a funny colour – she decided that this was confirmation of a terminal illness, and had images of herself emaciated and dying and her son being left all alone. The formulation was a revelation. She had not realised how much she was worried about dying and abandoning her son. Seeing how everything was linked together with anxiety meant that it had all started to make sense.

Employing CBT techniques

Careful consideration of details obtained from a diary may show a pattern of symptoms linked to specific events or anticipated events. It may also reveal how much preoccupation with diet there is and how restricted life has become. Pie charts can be constructed for symptoms such as abdominal pain, nausea and even rectal bleeding, particularly in those with irritable bowel syndrome. Using the pyramid technique things can be brought into proportion and space for more realistic interpretations may be opened up.

Checking and safety activities can be identified, such as frequent visits to the toilet 'just to be sure' to anticipate the fear of diarrhoea and incontinence, frequent self-examination, feeling the abdomen to look for lumps, frequent weighing to look for weight loss, checking on the internet, and the use of chat rooms even for proven problems, as for the health-anxious these can be alarmist. The demonstration that the symptoms from the Beck Anxiety Inventory overlap greatly with those when the patient experiences gastrointestinal symptoms can consolidate the association with anxiety. This realisation can be very helpful.

Patients can be asked to count the cost of the worry and preoccupation around their bowels, or their vomiting or fear of vomiting. This can then lead into consideration of the 'fear of disease' versus 'actually having the disease' model. They can be asked to look at the perceived awfulness of having bowel cancer or being incontinent on a trip out, then about the likelihood of this happening, particularly when considering the negative tests and the fact that they have never actually had 'an accident' before.

Jennifer was invited to keep a diary of her symptoms (nausea, vomiting and cough) and although it coincided with the week off medication leading up to the test (not an ideal time), she was surprised to find things had not been that bad, primarily as whenever she felt sick she had turned to the formulation. There was also a pattern linked to her son leaving for school and his return, which she immediately identified as 'very nerve racking' in case things had not gone well. She was proud of coping well, and now having identified a pattern following this discussion, her hacking cough, which was marked when she had first walked in, completely disappeared. At the end of the session this was remarked on, and she said perhaps that was because she was now much more relaxed. When asked whether she still felt sick, despite stopping the tablets, she was astonished to notice that the nausea had gone too – and that she felt hungry.

Behavioural experiments

Using the information obtained from the diary evaluation, the patient can be invited to test out some of the theories. These could include planning a trip out, gradually increasing the time spent away from home and gradually removing the need to find out where the toilets were in advance. Patients, particularly those with irritable bowel syndrome, may say that they have to go to the toilet many times in the morning and so can never leave the house at that time. It is worth considering that when at home they may not have tried to avoid excessive visits, and they used the toilet simply because they could.

For patients diagnosed with irritable bowel syndrome, a survey could be carried out among friends to see how much others suffered with 'wind' and 'feeling bloated', as these sensations are universal, so allowing this to be regarded as normal for the patient.

Patients obsessed with self-imposed dietary restrictions could test out whether these were really necessary in the light of the new anxiety model being embraced; this could then lead to a freeing up of lifestyle, rather than feeling 'trapped in' by their symptoms.

Common problems encountered in management

Some patients may have had an accident, in terms of incontinence, in a public situation, which has understandably unnerved them. Exploration of this event, special contributing factors and the likelihood of it happening again can be explored. It might, for example, have occurred prior to them starting treatment or have been related to something dietary which they could now avoid if they were planning to go out. Did anyone actually notice? What sensible precautions might they be able to take now? The anxiety equation (see Chapter 2, p. 9) can be a very helpful technique here, where you can build on the rescue and coping factors, as well as reducing the likelihood of it happening. If they struggle with this, ask them how they might advise a friend with a similar problem. This approach can help them think more clearly, freed from considering themselves in the particular situation.

The possibility of having to have an ileostomy or colostomy bag at some time in the future can be a very real problem, particularly in patients with inflammatory bowel disease. Again, the equation can be helpful here, as can a mini survey. For example, you might ask: 'In everyday life, with all those you encounter from day to day, have you ever been able to tell if someone has a bag or not?'. Seeing and handling an actual bag, with explanation from a specialist nurse, or meeting a patient who has one, can help demystify it all and make it seem less of a threat.

CHAPTER 13

Endocrinology

Patients in endocrinology clinics with health anxiety

Clarifying past medical communications

Endocrinology clinics, as well as assessing and treating the very common problems of diabetes and thyroid disease (which can of course coexist with health anxiety), also admit patients with non-specific symptoms such as dizziness and fatigue, for which no obvious cause can be found. Of these patients with medically unexplained symptoms, many will have had a myriad of investigations, some of which may have been found to be mildly abnormal, fuelling further concern.

Patients with 'brittle' diabetes, with frequent hypoglycaemic attacks, are an interesting group in their own right. They frequently have anxiety of emotional origin and without treatment that addresses this, they have a poor prognosis (Tattersall *et al*, 1991). See Case example 13.1.

Case example 13.1: Diabetes with health anxiety

Sue, a 22-year-old woman, had diabetes. She lived at home with her mum and a 5-year-old daughter, and her long-standing partner lived with his parents nearby. Sue and her partner had no plans to move in with each other. She experienced chronic fatigue. She had missed a lot of schooling through this, and although quite bright, had performed badly in examinations. She had had a number of 'hypos' (episodes of hypoglycaemia) recently, mainly at night when she made a strange noise that woke her mother up. She was too scared of collapsing to take her daughter to school and was terrified that she was going to die in the near future, which had led to her leading a very restricted and isolated lifestyle. Her partner, who was unemployed, took their daughter to school and picked her up every day, but he resented this and their relationship was becoming increasingly acrimonious. She had been admitted many times to hospital as an emergency; in some of these cases her blood sugar had been found to be low and at other times she had some symptoms of hypoglycaemia when in fact her blood sugar had been normal. This was very confusing for her and left her feeling out of control. In addition, hospital staff had inferred that she should always err on the side of caution and contact the emergency services if in any doubt.

Evaluating and interpreting symptoms

It can be difficult for doctors to evaluate non-specific symptoms where there is a history of diabetes, or possible autoimmune disease, and thus patients can be given mixed messages, those of the emergency staff at times conflicting with those of the routine clinical team. Health-anxious patients are likely to err on the side of caution and inconsistent advice can be very troubling.

In endocrinology, making a diary is especially important. It delivers a record of what is going on in what is often a confusing state of affairs. Patterns can be elicited which can give a sense of confidence over times when the patient needs to worry, and also other times when they can have more confidence that in fact all is well. At times when they are just not feeling up to scratch or exhibiting symptoms of anxiety, the recognition that many of the endocrine symptoms overlap with anxiety can be especially helpful.

In all the confusion that can arise, important medical points can be missed. Sometimes, a reminder that all people with diabetes with a history of hypoglycaemia need to carry around a supply of glucose, with a rehash of the warning signs of hypoglycaemia, is needed.

Developing a formulation

The formulation for Sue centred around a recent encounter with her partner when he brought their daughter back from school to her house. They had an argument over whether she should be allowed to play (Sue's preference) or whether she should sort out her school bag and eat her tea first. He had appeared fed up with looking after her and wanted some time to himself. They usually had tea together, but it could be a strain, and tea was not ready on that day. Sue noticed that she was beginning to feel dizzy and her head hurt; she also felt nauseated and concluded that she was getting a hypo, so she asked her partner to call an ambulance. She thought, 'Here we go again, I'll never get any better, what if I collapse now and Nolly (her daughter) sees me die'. She had images of herself being buried and others of Nolly growing up without her, living with her partner and his parents and being terribly unhappy. Sue lay on the sofa and started to check her pulse, which she thought was getting fainter, and thought that her skin was turning a funny colour. She was terrified, thought she was going to collapse and felt a complete failure.

When the ambulance arrived, the medical attendants checked her blood sugar, which was normal, but as a precaution they took her to accident and emergency. As in the past, her partner and mother had to placate Nolly and look after her until Sue returned with the all-clear a few hours later.

Employing CBT techniques

The formulation had highlighted Sue's lack of control over the situation and her feelings of being a failure. She felt hopeless. When situations around health anxiety and symptoms seem completely muddled, it is a good first step to get the patient to complete a diary of all the events. Some factual evidence to clarify what were recurring, potentially life-threatening situations was paramount here. Everybody involved was uncertain what was going on, erring (understandably) on the side of caution and universally feeling dissatisfied. The therapist asked Sue to keep a fairly detailed diary of events, general activity and feelings, but in addition constructed one retrospectively. This was documenting the timing of accident and emergency attendances and the outcome: hypoglycaemia *v.* no hypoglycaemia, and whether or not Sue was admitted to hospital, and for how long.

Interpretation of the (quite detailed) retrospective diary revealed an interesting scenario. Very few of Sue's contacts with accident and emergency revealed any medical problem, and the few that did were exclusively nocturnal. The prospective diary revealed an association of symptoms with stressful interactions with her mother and partner, usually concerning what Sue wanted for Nolly. It also revealed how limited her activities were and how isolated she had become.

At these times Sue also scored highly on the Beck Anxiety Inventory, and she was asked to consider whether fear was a large part of the problem. In addition, the formulation highlighted her sense of failure.

She was invited to take a bit more control over her life, in terms of decision-making for her daughter, with some protected time for the two of them to play together after school. She also felt that the teatime meal had become an ordeal when her partner was there, and in fact it turned out that he was not that bothered about eating with her and Nolly, but just did it out of a sense of duty. After some encouragement, Sue was asked to consider whether she could do some of the school runs herself.

Sue, when she did go out, which was never very far, perhaps just to the corner shop or the supermarket with her Mum, never took a supply of glucose with her, nor did she wear a medical bracelet to alert others to her condition if she collapsed. Re-training by the diabetic nurse in recognition of the warning signs of hypoglycaemia, along with review of her medication and a recognition of when the serious problems tended to occur (at night, and helped by increasing calorie intake before bed) helped enormously. She was able to begin to make sense of what was going on and what she could do to help. She began to grow in confidence and felt less tired, and eventually was encouraged to consider making the bus journey to pick up Nolly from school.

Behavioural experiments

Discussion of Sue's fears of collapse centred around the use of the anxiety equation: it was *unlikely* she would collapse, and although in that unlikely event she might feel embarrassed, she was invited to consider how would she feel towards someone who was unexpectedly taken ill in a public place. She also concluded there were coping and rescue factors she could employ, such as carrying the glucose when she went out as a routine, letting someone know where she was going, purchasing a mobile phone, letting the school and a few of the other mums know about her diabetes and her fears. She also realised how much fun it would be for Nolly to have Mum pick her up (Dad still took Nolly to school as Sue remained quite tired in the mornings).

Eventually, she managed the school pick up herself, initially with her partner there for moral support and later on her own. She made a friend in another mum in whom she confided some of her problems. There were no adverse events, and as her confidence rose, the management of her diabetes fell into place. As her fears reduced, she began to set longer-term goals for herself: attending night school 2 days a week and possibly enrolling for a part-time college course the following year. She and her partner also faced up to the fact that their relationship was not going anywhere and the best thing to do would be to just remain friends. Sue felt as if a huge burden had been lifted off her and slowly her fatigue began to ease.

Common problems encountered in management

In endocrinology, fatigue tends to be a very common problem and care must be taken to consider whether depression is part of the problem. Of course, this may be the case in other specialties too and is discussed in Chapter 9. Screening for depression with simple instruments can help to clarify this and identify depression, so that CBT can be more appropriately directed or antidepressant medication may be introduced.

With patients whose anxiety is caused by unstable diabetes, it is worth making sure that they understand their condition properly, and it may well be necessary to liaise with their specialist nurse. Some patients fail to understand properly the requirements of diet and carbohydrate intake, even if they appear to know what they are doing; misunderstandings are common.

CHAPTER 14

Neurology

Neurological conditions and health anxiety

Health anxiety is especially common in neurology patients – one in four has the condition, a higher proportion than in other medical clinics (Tyrer *et al*, 2011*a*). Patients may just be offered a single appointment to exclude a more serious problem but they often have frequent investigations and when tests come back negative for underlying pathology, they tend not to be offered help for their anxiety.

Some of the most commonly feared conditions in health-anxious individuals are neurological illnesses such as brain tumours and multiple sclerosis (MS). Headaches are common in all people but frequently considered by the health-anxious patient to be evidence of a primary brain tumour or cerebral secondary deposits. Multiple sclerosis is often feared as it too is relatively common and the presenting symptoms are varied, tend to come and go (although not as frequently as health-anxious patients tend to believe) and accurate diagnosis is difficult. The symptoms of headache, perceived memory loss, clumsiness, twitching, involuntary movements, blurred vision, depersonalisation (the feeling of being unreal), dizziness and feeling faint, tingling in the extremities and trembling, are all common symptoms of anxiety but can also be part of neurological disease. They are frequently difficult to evaluate, and in many cases patients are overinvestigated for possible conditions such as Parkinson's disease.

Epilepsy is also a common condition and, as seizures can take many forms, sometimes this may be considered in anxious patients who experience depersonalisation – a distressing phenomenon where the patient feels as if they are detached from their surroundings, often accompanied by derealisation, the feeling that the surroundings too are strange. If this occurs frequently or is powerful enough, it may lead the clinician to suspect epilepsy.

Clarifying past medical communications

Multiple sclerosis is often considered as a differential diagnosis for non-specific neurological symptoms, and mentioning it in passing as a possible diagnosis can be extraordinarily worrying for patients, especially as in the early stages it can be difficult to confirm or refute. Patients worried by this can interpret every bodily sensation or change as evidence confirming the diagnosis. They frequently search on the internet for clues, and as the condition is so varied, they can easily find things to fit with their presumed pathology (Case example 14.1).

Case example 14.1: Dizziness after meningitis

Zoe, a dancer, had experienced a debilitating episode of viral meningitis, which had led to a brief hospital admission and some time off work. When she started to improve enough to begin some gentle training, she suffered a mild exacerbation of her symptoms, with some dizziness and fatigue. When she went back to her doctor for a check-up, he mentioned that it was almost certainly going to settle down but added that if it did not, it might just mean that there was some other condition underlying it. Zoe went home distraught and immediately started looking up the causes of dizziness and headaches on the internet. She concluded that she probably already had evidence of a brain tumour, as she recalled that she occasionally had a bit of blurred vision, and sometimes she experienced slight tingling in her fingers and around her mouth, all of which indicated to her that the 'tumour' was spreading.

Evaluating and interpreting symptoms

Clarification of non-specific symptoms in neurology can be difficult, especially in primary care. As a result, insistent patients may often be referred at an early stage to exclude more serious pathology. In the case above, Zoe continued to feel unwell, noticing additional problems such as feeling she was a bit weaker on one side when she was training. Eventually, she went back to see another doctor at the surgery, ostensibly to get some more medication, but in reality it was to get a second opinion. She was, however, too nervous to mention her fears about her brain tumour, but did stress her blurring of vision. She tentatively mentioned some of the other symptoms she had been experiencing but the doctor just put them down to resuming her training. Briefly reassured, Zoe decided she had resumed her exercise programme too soon and decided to have a few days resting. She began to feel depressed and withdrawn, and spent more and more time again on the internet. When she did eventually leave home to go to the supermarket, all she was able to see were others with some form of disability or in wheelchairs, and, feeling increasingly distressed, she rapidly purchased a few items and went home.

Zoe's visits to the GP became increasingly frequent, but she still failed to voice all her fears. Still, she did ask whether she could have further tests. Eventually she was referred to an ophthalmologist, who could find no underlying problems and she was strongly reassured. But the benefits of this were only temporary. She could accept that the blurring of vision was nothing to do with her eyes, but that meant to her it was more likely to be due to an underlying brain tumour.

Developing a formulation

For Zoe, the formulation was based on a recent day when she was training specifically for a new audition in an attempt to get back to full-time work (she was currently working freelance). She became convinced that the left side of her body was a bit weaker than the right and her headache became worse. She became terrified and tried gripping things with both hands to compare the strength on each side, after which she began to feel that she could hardly move at all, and her hands started tingling. She scrutinised herself closely in the exercise mirror and thought that her face was twitching. She felt she now had incontrovertible evidence of a brain tumour with accompanying epilepsy. She knew this meant that her dancing career was at an end, and not only that, but she would never get another job. She would end up crippled in a wheelchair and had images of herself dying emaciated in hospital.

Employing CBT techniques

The formulation highlighted to Zoe how terrified she was feeling and how important her dancing was to her. Linking her symptoms to periods of training when she was anxious about her performance, and to other symptoms of anxiety as in the Beck Anxiety Inventory, illustrated a clear pattern. When she was chatting with friends or actually performing in a show, they were not present, and both Zoe and her therapist concluded that symptoms were unlikely to discriminate anxiety from a tumour in this way. She was then asked to consider that she might have 'fear of' a brain tumour rather than 'actually having' one.

Consideration was also given to addressing her selective attention to comments that her doctors had made, and how information on the internet might produce bias.

Behavioural experiments

Zoe was invited to carry out an experiment around her checking behaviour. She was asked to perform all her checking behaviours for 2 days while measuring her anxiety throughout the day (these included comparing her strength on both sides, checking her body for asymmetry and checking on the internet), but then to avoid any of these activities for the rest of the week, while continuing to rate her level of worry. Zoe completed the task fairly well, although found it difficult, especially about checking in the mirror. Her anxiety was very high for the first 2 days, then rose even higher on the day she had to stop checking, as she found it hard to stop. It then gradually reduced, apart from one day when it rose dramatically. After discussion she remembered that on the day when it peaked again she had read an article in the paper about a dancer who had developed a rare progressive neurological disease and died within a year. She had felt a bit better the following day when she rationalised to herself that this condition was rare and not related to a brain tumour.

Zoe had to use her mirror for dance practice, and although she tried hard, it was a challenge for her to realise (really for the first time) that her body was not entirely symmetrical, and she was troubled by this. Her therapist asked her to consider whether anyone was completely identical on both sides; she was not sure but said that on balance she thought she was odd in this way. Together with her therapist they did a survey of their friends, asking specifically for various areas of the body and whether they were identical on both sides, for example, skin markings, facial features, breast size in women, feet and so on. It transpired that no one was completely the same on both sides. It was a revelation to Zoe.

For health-anxious patients with a particularly troublesome symptom such as headache, when each headache seems to indicate incontrovertible evidence of a brain tumour (even if they have had the same headache on and off for years), the techniques of the pie chart and the pyramid are especially helpful (see Chapter 5). For the pie chart, the therapist and the patient might construct together a list of all the causes of headache, including as many innocuous ones as possible. The list would be likely to contain brain tumour (the patient's first thought), migraine, flu, a cold, viral infections, hunger, stress, hangover, medication, fatigue including a very late night, or not sleeping. The patient is then asked to consider everyone in the local supermarket (for example) who has a headache today and work out the percentage for each category, starting with the most common first; as the pie chart is completed, there is virtually no room left for the brain tumour. This helps to get the important message across that not every headache means a brain tumour! This can be a huge revelation to patients.

Zoe had become increasingly preoccupied by every little ache, pain and tingling sensation, or little involuntary movements such as her eyelid twitching. When she noticed anything she had an overwhelming urge to visit the doctor or ask one of her friends what they thought it was for reassurance. She agreed that the doctor would probably dismiss a twitch in a finger if it had only been present for a day, and so she was asked to use the technique of 'listing symptoms'. Zoe and the therapist agreed between them that you could probably leave a symptom about 10 days before seeking advice, by writing the symptom down on a piece of paper and putting the date for 10 days' time next to it, and not checking on that symptom again until then. By doing this, you were not ignoring it, you were simply evaluating it more appropriately. Zoe managed this, initially showing the therapist the list, but later keeping some things to herself, a manoeuvre suggested by the therapist as Zoe became more confident in using the technique. Eventually, minor symptoms/sensations could still be present on the list 10 days later, but she could choose to ignore them.

Common problems encountered in management

One of the most difficult aspects of investigation for patients in neurological clinics is that testing is not always clear-cut, and many tests, such as brain scans and lumbar puncture, are unpleasant. The tests may be inconclusive or expensive (e.g. magnetic resonance imaging scans) and a 'wait-and-see' policy needs to be adopted in some cases. This wait can be intolerable for the health-anxious patient. As so many of the diagnoses in neurology are uncertain, with frequent follow-up appointments needed to clarify alternative diagnoses, the combination of worry about serious illness, debilitating handicap and devastating suffering can be reinforced on every occasion (Case example 14.2).

Case example 14.2: Fear of stroke

Paul, aged 34, worked as a medical photographer in a large teaching hospital. He had been married for 8 years and had two children, a son of 8 and a daughter of 4. Paul described himself as having always been a worrier. His mum and dad split up when he was 7, and to him this event had happened out of the blue when overnight he and his mum went to stay with his mum's aunt at the other end of the country. He lost touch with all his friends and was systematically bullied at his new school for several years until they moved back. The worries about his health began when he was 21. A friend at university suffered a minor stroke following a blood clot from a previously undiagnosed 'hole in the heart'. The fact that someone of his own age could have a neurological condition had scared him, and from time to time he began to notice some tingling in his arms. Around the time of his final exams he noticed the tingling increase and he also began to feel dizzy at times. He visited his GP who felt that there was probably little wrong, but said he would like to see Paul again if the symptoms persisted.

Paul monitored his symptoms continuously and was increasingly alarmed, as they were present for most of the time. He was convinced that he too was going to develop a stroke, so he purchased a blood pressure machine. After recording his blood pressure he was alarmed, as it seemed to vary enormously and at times was raised. On returning to see his GP, the decision was made to refer him to a specialist, mainly to exclude the possibility of multiple sclerosis and to put Paul's mind at rest.

Paul was devastated at the possibility of having multiple sclerosis. He immediately searched the condition on the internet, exploring all the other features of the disease. He became convinced that he was also developing other neurological manifestations such as partial numbness in his fingers and arms when waking from sleep, and at times he thought his vision was blurred. By the time he saw the neurologist, he was absolutely convinced he had multiple sclerosis. To his astonishment the specialist was not at all convinced and arranged some preliminary investigations which suggested little evidence of the illness, and once more a follow-up appointment was made to reassess the problem 1 month later.

Paul was consumed with anxiety. He struggled through his exams and then seemed to go to pieces, visiting his GP repeatedly to get some reassurance or treatment. Unable to see the same doctor at each visit, he received conflicting opinions about the possible diagnosis. When he eventually received the follow-up neurology appointment, he was told it was exceedingly unlikely that he had multiple sclerosis and so he should stop worrying. Although relieved by this news on the day, by the next day all his fears had returned, and having been discharged from further follow-up he had no clue about which way to turn.

After a year of worry, Paul met a new girlfriend and for a while his fears receded and he felt happier and more settled. The couple started living together, and when she became pregnant they made plans to marry. Then, one morning, he noticed a slight tremor in his right index finger, and with increasing horror he realised that the neurologist was probably right, in that he did not have multiple sclerosis, as the diagnosis was really that of Parkinson's disease. The internet checking began again in earnest and he started to notice difficulties in concentration at work, which became, in his mind, evidence of developing Parkinsonian dementia. Repeated visits to his GP failed to reassure him and he was re-referred to the neurologist. He was told that there was no evidence of Parkinson's disease and discharged.

After the initial excitement of the pregnancy, Paul became convinced that he would be a cripple before the child grew up, and continued to be obsessed with every minor bodily sensation. He checked his body and his mental functioning repeatedly, including trying to memorise lists and pestering his girlfriend and other family members for reassurance, sometimes infuriating them with his incessant questions. He sought private neurological appointments with several different neurologists, using up his meagre savings in the process. Although he put a brave face on things, the wedding day was clouded for him by the prospect of a life as a cripple, accompanied by feelings of irresponsibility and guilt.

For the past 8 years he had been plagued by anxiety, he tried a long course of sertaline to little effect, as his doctor felt there were also features of depression at times. To compound his problems, he experienced an episode of viral labyrinthitis. This was treated with a combination of medication that induced iatrogenic akathisia (involuntary movements that can be suppressed, to some extent consciously), which he found incredibly distressing. He interpreted this side-effect as further evidence that he was susceptible to what had now become a whole range of neurological conditions, with Parkinson's disease the most likely. At times, his anxiety necessitated brief admissions to the local psychiatric unit where witnessing the extrapyramidal side-effects of patients taking high doses of antipsychotic medication terrified him further.

The formulation at the beginning of therapy for an episode of tingling in his arm when he was very anxious was that he would end up with a severe progressive neurological condition, where he could not keep still and would lose the ability to control any of his bodily functions. He imagined his wife and children being disgusted and abandoning him, so that he would have to face the rest of his life alone.

He and his therapist considered jointly which factors were helping to maintain his fear and identified all his complex ways of checking, such as moving his arm into a range of positions to check whether it induced weakness or tingling, and counting all the times he had to go to pass urine to see whether he was losing control over his bladder. He also made long lists of how to perform various tasks, and then felt he had to memorise them in order to, for example, get in and out of the car, and sometimes this extended to feeling that he had forgotten how to drive. This exercise also identified the extent of his reassurance-seeking, as in addition to beleaguering family and work colleagues, he visited the GP at least once a week, and was a frequent user of the out-of-hours service.

He tried an experiment in which he was asked to examine the effects of checking excessively on some days and on others when he was asked to resist all checking. He was also asked to stop making lists. He found, rather to his surprise, a degree of relief on the days that he did not check. He was encouraged to record on a piece of paper all those symptoms that troubled him with the date they appeared, and negotiated with his therapist at fixed agreed times (rather than rushing to the doctor) the reassessment of the problem and whether it was still present and warranted further attention. These exercises were very difficult for him and he frequently gave in to the desire to check or ring up the doctor. He was asked to keep a diary to tease out relationships between his safety-seeking behaviours and his anxiety, but he found this quite difficult. His therapist measured his progress by getting him to rate his beliefs about illnesses at each visit, and by helping him to recognise triggers, initially retrospectively and then anticipating them for the week ahead.

For some reason, he remained excessively anxious every morning. When considering this in more detail, he mentioned that he hated his mother telephoning at about 8 every morning just as he was leaving for work to see how he was feeling. He hated telling her he was still worried and found it very difficult not to disclose any symptoms and ask for reassurance. His mother also tended to be anxious and as she lived alone, he felt he was adding to her problems. Following discussion, he made an arrangement (under the pretext of being rushed for work and getting the children to school) to telephone her three times a week at a time more suited to him, which he could vary. He established a pattern of speaking to her when he felt less anxious, and asking about her own feelings first. To his relief and surprise, this fairly simple move produced a dramatic reduction in his anxiety.

CHAPTER 15

Genitourinary medicine

Health-anxious patients in genitourinary clinics

Genitourinary medicine is as much about prevention of infection as it is about its detection and treatment. Patients who may have put themselves at risk of infection are encouraged to come forward for testing as many sexually transmitted infections, especially in the early stages, may be asymptomatic. Usually, there is a delay between contracting a sexually transmitted infection (STI) and the relevant test becoming positive. This can be as short as up to 2 weeks for gonorrhoea and chlamydia, and as long as 3 months for HIV and syphilis. So a patient attending for a check-up 3 weeks after an episode of unprotected sex, with negative screening, including that for HIV and syphilis, will have to re-attend 9 weeks later for the blood tests to be completed. This can be a very anxious time, particularly if they are in another relationship, as during this time they should practise safe sex or abstain.

There still remains a degree of stigma around sexual health and this can make it hard, if not impossible, for patients to talk about their worries with others, and very often this extends to health professionals too. In addition, unlike most other diseases that people fear, such as cancer, there is the issue of transmission and guilt is often a major issue that needs to be addressed in therapy. What is more, all this occurs within the context of intimate relationships, where trust can be seriously undermined and relationships potentially permanently damaged. Occasionally, test results can be equivocal and need repeating, and occasionally false–positive and false–negative results may be obtained. One person in a couple may test positive for an infection, but their partner may not, further adding to the confusion.

There is also the question of confidentiality and partner notification (contact tracing for the partners of infection). Patients are given clinic numbers and these, coupled with the patient's date of birth, are used to replace names on all biological specimens. You are not allowed to discuss any aspect of a patient's care with their partner unless they have given their express permission (ideally, clearly documented and signed). This can cause frustration for patients, even if you explain that it is official legislation and that you would be breaking the law, but there are ways of couching these issues in sensitive terms, so patients feel listened to and understood.

This legislation is in place to give people the confidence to come forward for confidential testing to help prevent the spread of infection, so it is also very much a public health issue. For example, if a patient is found to have gonorrhoea, but is adamant that they, for whatever reason, cannot tell their partner to come in to the clinic for a check-up, this can be done for them without revealing their name, although the precise nature of the infection cannot be specifically discussed.

Genitourinary medicine staff are familiar with these issues and well trained to deal with them, but they can be unnerving to anyone unfamiliar with the specialty, and some advice may need to be sought.

Clarifying past medical communications

Over the past three decades, with the emergence of HIV infection, there has been huge publicity around all sexually transmitted infections. Sometimes, these have taken the form of high-profile campaigns such as the HIV publicity in the 1980s. To the health-anxious patient this publicity can heighten their concern, and has led to many patients of all ages with a negligible possibility of having contracted HIV coming into clinics for repeated testing. To compound their fears, testing for HIV was less accurate at the start of the outbreak, and the window period between exposure to infection and the longest time it took for a blood test to become positive was less certain, with reports ranging up to 2 years. More recently, probably as a result of increased migration, the incidence of syphilis has increased, with a corresponding increase in worry about contracting this in health-anxious individuals.

Fears of these two conditions and other STIs continue to plague the health anxious in these clinics. There has also been heightened publicity around ovarian cancer and how it tends to present late and with non-specific symptoms that can mimic other conditions such as irritable bowel syndrome. Similarly, prostatic cancer has been much publicised, and these two conditions can be a major concern for slightly older patients attending genitourinary medicine clinics.

By their nature, genitourinary medicine/sexual health clinics are easily accessible. Patients do not need to be referred by their GP. In addition, they are not sectorised, so anybody can attend any clinic in the country. Many departments have 'walk-in clinics' too, some with same-day HIV testing, so the opportunity for repeated testing, even if not clinically indicated, is enormous and in the patient's hands. The records for clinics are not centralised and it is accepted that some patients give false names and addresses through fear of disclosure. This kind of open access serves the public health nature of the service well, but can compound the problem for those who are health anxious.

Evaluating and interpreting symptoms

Symptoms can be extraordinarily various in both HIV and syphilis, and as many are related to immune deficiency in HIV, a number of fearful patients become obsessed with every cough or cold, attributing these to evidence of impaired immunity. Patients become hooked on repeat testing, 'just to put my mind at rest, doctor', but the reassurance does not last and the fears return. In addition, waiting for the result can be an extremely anxious time. Patients can become extremely hypervigilant and because of the fears around transmission, may scrutinise their partners for signs of disease as well. See Case example 15.1.

Case example 15.1: Chlamydia and health anxiety

Gordon was a senior manager with a big company and happily married with two teenage sons. During one Christmas time he had a brief 'fling' and unprotected sex with an attractive junior girl in an adjoining office. He regretted it, felt a bit stupid and tried to put it behind him. He was, however, feeling a bit guilty and mentioned it to a work colleague who was also a good friend. The colleague teased Gordon about it saying that everyone knew she 'slept around'. Gordon felt mortified and full of fear. He did not know much about STIs and had never been to a genitourinary medicine clinic, but he had recently read an article on chlamydia saying how common it was, and that it could have serious complications, particularly for women. He felt terrible, sick and anxious, and overwhelmed with guilt. He did not know what to do next. Eventually, he went to the lavatory, and in a cubicle minutely examined his genitalia for signs of disease. He was not sure what to look for other than a penile discharge, but he noticed a mark on the penis that he had never seen before. He was filled with panic and on going back to his desk, looked up chlamydia and other STIs on the internet. To his horror he saw that rashes could be a manifestation of all sorts of conditions, but also that chlamydia could be present without any symptoms. He began to feel unwell with palpitations and stomach cramps and had to go home early.

The conviction that he had chlamydia grew rapidly. It had been a month since the sexual encounter, and he and his wife had made love many times since, without a condom as his wife had a coil fitted. He could not contemplate having sex again, especially without a condom, but had no excuse to use one. His health anxiety grew and he began to check his body and monitor his wife's health all the time. He developed strange sensations when he passed urine and had problems achieving an erection. He noticed his joints ached at times and his stomach pains became worse, and he became convinced that he had developed a particular complication of chlamydial infection, Reiter's syndrome, where joint aches and pains are the main symptoms. He could not bring himself to attend a genitourinary medicine clinic, so went repeatedly to his GP. He did not mention his fears, and the doctor performed more and more tests, but it did not occur to him to do a swab for chlamydia. As the routine blood tests came back negative, Gordon was initially reassured, but the worries always returned and he would go back to see the GP, who eventually referred him to a gastroenterologist. Here he was investigated for a possible peptic ulcer, but the gastroscopy was negative. Gordon was devastated, to him this was categorical evidence that he had a complicated chlamydial infection.

He took the plunge and booked into a genitourinary medicine clinic. He informed them that he had had chlamydia for a year and needed treatment. He confessed about the brief affair and underwent testing. He had to wait a week for the results, which were all negative, but he did not believe that, thinking his results might have been confused with those of someone else. He went back 2 weeks later and saw another doctor who repeated the tests. The results were once again negative. Gordon did not know what to do. The doctors would not give him antibiotics, and moreover had announced that unless he had unprotected sex again he was all-clear and they would do nothing further.

He contacted a genitourinary medicine clinic in another town and had a further set of tests. When the results were negative again he broke down, and after discussion the doctor referred him for psychological help to a colleague who practised CBT.

Developing a formulation with specific examples

The formulation for Gordon was centred around a Thursday evening after work, when he and his wife were watching TV. She mentioned that her psoriasis was flaring up a bit and that she also had a bit of toothache. Gordon began to feel very sick and anxious and looked across at her. He thought she looked a bit pale and he immediately concluded that the chlamydial infection he was convinced he had given her had led to her developing Reiter's syndrome. He felt this had lowered the ability of her immune system to deal with infection and so her toothache was a manifestation of this. He had visions of her finding out too late that he had given her the infection and leaving him. He imagined that he would never see his sons again and would end up living a life of fear on his own. At the heart of Gordon's fear was the prospect of living alone, with a chronic illness, completely alienated from his family. He was also consumed with guilt as he was convinced he had ruined his wife's life too.

Another case concerned Tina (Case example 15.2).

Case example 15.2: Fear of AIDS

Tina was a young woman who had spent a year travelling with her friend to the Far East. They had ended their trip in Thailand, where she had fallen in love with a young Thai man called Johnny. After returning back to the UK, she arranged for Johnny to visit and they made long-term plans to live together. They thought through all the practicalities and Johnny returned to Thailand to make the arrangements. His family were very supportive as they had met Tina and liked her very much, and felt they would make a good match. He also promised to try to send some money back home to Thailand. At first things went well and they were very happy. Tina was a financial adviser and was soon back in work with her old company. She earned a good salary and, although Johnny was not able to get work, Tina did not mind. They had talked about marriage, but Johnny seemed a little reluctant.

After a few months, however, Johnny became unwell. He was tired, had lost weight and developed a cough. He insisted that he wanted to go back to Thailand to his family. Tina was very concerned and flew back with him, but had to return to work after a week, although she had made arrangements to take some leave at the end of the month. She left some money with him and arranged for him to attend the hospital for some investigations. She never saw him again. He deteriorated fast and died 2 weeks later of pneumonia.

Tina was devastated and immediately flew back to Thailand. She arranged to see Johnny's doctor who explained to her that Johnny's death was almost certainly related to HIV infection and subsequent AIDS, but they would never know for sure as he had refused to have a test. He was very kind and arranged for Tina to have an HIV test, which was negative. She was advised to have another in a couple of months. In fact, Tina and Johnny had rarely had sex without a condom, and they had not had any sexual contact over the previous month because of his illness. Back in the UK, Tina felt lost and vulnerable. She felt she could not tell her family what Johnny had died of as they would be disapproving and worry a lot, and she did not want his memory sullied. She was grieving for him, and missing him terribly, but also felt angry with him for not having the test and not confiding more in her. She felt sure that he had probably suspected he was HIV-positive. She suspected that he had many girlfriends in the past.

Tina returned to work and almost immediately developed a nasty throat infection. She remembered about the repeat HIV test and was convinced she had AIDS and was going to die. A second HIV test was negative but she was advised to repeat it again in a month, when she would be outside the window period. Meanwhile, she continued to worry and dredged the internet for information. She became more and more alarmed and began to drink heavily. She started noticing all sorts of aches and pains, felt she had more coughs and colds than usual and developed epigastric pain, which she began to think was cancer, somehow related to the HIV. She continued to have more HIV tests, which were all negative, but she never believed the results. She became withdrawn, only going out to work, and had turned down a few potentially lucrative jobs as she could not see the point in working when she was going to die. Her doctor eventually referred her to a general physician but no cause for her problem was found.

When eventually she was identified as health anxious and began receiving CBT, she was also quite depressed. A formulation was made of a recent Saturday morning when she woke up with a headache and epigastric pain. She remembered drinking half a bottle of whisky the night before. Then she remembered Johnny and began to cry; she felt guilty that she had not been there for him when he died, imagined him gasping for breath with pneumonia and crying out for her. She then started imagining her own death, who would come to the funeral, and worried she had not done anything much with her life and had no children to live on after her. She went into the bathroom, looked in the mirror and saw a patient with terminal AIDS staring back at her. She started checking her skin for rashes and prodded her abdomen until it became extremely sore. She went into the kitchen and by the door saw another letter from Thailand, from Johnny's family asking for money. She felt sick, then became very angry and wished she had never gone travelling. The conclusion was that she felt she had been used and that she had wasted her life.

Employing CBT techniques

After taking the history, looking at all the symptoms and what they meant for Gordon, and constructing the formulation, the therapist decided to draw a pie chart for the causes of toothache (Gordon's wife's complaint). It did not take long to realise that there was definitely no room for chlamydia! They also established that most of the symptoms he noticed were only present when he was trying to relax in the evening and ruminating about his fears. Many checking behaviours were identified, especially over-observing his wife and her psoriasis, the severity of which he linked to the chlamydia fear too.

They also discussed at some length the merits of disclosing to his wife what he had done. He would be able to get rid of some of his guilt, but she would have to deal with the fact that he had had what he considered to be a stupid, meaningless liaison, and the lack of trust that would follow could take years to rebuild, if at all. He also felt that there was a good chance she might leave him. After several conversations around this, he decided to stick with the psychological therapy and work hard at it for her as well as himself. He wanted to see whether he could come to terms with the problem and eradicate the fear. He could then make the most of the rest of their years together.

The approach with Tina was to consider and validate her mixed feelings about Johnny. She began to understand things from his point of view, but equally to accept that it was OK to feel upset about some of the decisions he had made. She and the therapist had a discussion about the transmission rates for HIV in different situations and this helped her to put the problem into perspective. A diary of symptoms and activities showed that many of them, especially the epigastric pain and low mood, were linked to the excessive amount of alcohol she was drinking at weekends. It also revealed how little exercise she had taken and how unfit she had become. She was asked to consider that as there was a strong possibility that she did not have HIV, would it do any harm to try to get fitter?

She was very troubled by the letters from Johnny's family in Thailand, asking for money. She was worried about them, but could not afford to send them any further funds. On discussion, she and the therapist worked out that Johnny's family were no worse off than the average family. They also concluded that they may have assumed she was wealthier than was the case. The letters were also a constant reminder of Johnny's death. Tina decided to write to them explaining that she had been pleased to help them but could no longer afford to do so. She explained that the cost of living in the UK was very high and she was not always able to find work. Once she had sent the letter, she felt a huge weight lifted off her. She also started to feel better about Johnny. She found out some photographs of them both together, which she had hidden away, and displayed them again.

She was encouraged to set some goals. The first short-term goal was to go back to getting fit again, and so returned to the fitness club where she was previously a member. She felt a great deal better back with her old friends in the club.

Behavioural experiments

Gordon was invited to experiment with cessation of checking and to measure how that affected his anxiety. It was going to be difficult as much of the checking had become a habit, and he and the therapist had to work out carefully between them how to look at his wife without making a quick check. One technique for this was to consider that everyone looked a bit different at various times of the day and from day to day, and it was only if there was a protracted deterioration or change that he should feel alarmed. So Gordon could expect his wife's appearance to vary. Also, if he noticed something new about her such as a spot on her face, he was not to keep looking at it. It was decided he should adopt the 'listing symptoms' approach and only check it 10–14 days later.

In fact, Gordon found the exercise easier than he had expected and limiting the checking provided some relief. He even went out for a meal with his wife and forgot about the problem completely, something he had not done for over a year. He also noticed that some of his symptoms had lessened and he needed less antacids for his indigestion. He was invited to consider the evidence that he might be 'worried about' carrying and passing on chlamydia rather than 'actually having' it. He was doing well, finding confirmatory evidence for himself, and he had even resumed fairly normal sexual relations with his wife (although part of him thought they might as well have sex as the damage was done). Then they went on a walking holiday in Wales. It was a spur-of-the-moment decision and in part reflected the fact that Gordon was feeling a lot better. Neither of them was particularly fit, however, and after the first day, and for the rest of the week, they both suffered a lot of joint pains. Rather than thinking that this might be par for the course, Gordon felt it must be due to Reiter's syndrome and all his fears returned with a vengeance. A re-evaluation of the likely cause of the pains, how they were worse after more strenuous activity, and that some of the other walkers they met who did this as a regular activity suffered too, enabled him to see things in proportion. He was disappointed with the setback though and had lost some confidence. He still had some niggling doubts and felt he should have some more tests.

The therapist asked two questions: first, had the testing ever helped in the past (to which the answer was no, because in the long term he had never accepted the results), and second, what was the cost of continuing to worry? They made a list of the cost. It made poor reading: depressed and anxious for the rest of his life, a deterioration of his marriage, an inability to enjoy the future of his sons, and a constant preoccupation with his self. The list made Gordon feel extraordinarily depressed and hopeless. The therapist then asked him to consider what he would feel like if he chose to change, to challenge his worries and ultimately leave them behind. What would he really like to achieve in life, what would he like to be remembered for?

This list was quite different. He was encouraged to think back to plans he and his wife had made in the past: what they would do when the children left home, how they would spend their time when they had a bit more money, what they would do to the house and where they would travel. Gordon's mood began to lift as he made the list, and at the end he was reminded by the therapist about the cognitive theory of emotion, simplified to 'how you think affects how you feel'.

125

Gordon was invited to set some short-term and longer-term goals, and with the new list in front of him this was surprisingly easy. He re-engaged with therapy, resisted the tests, made plans for the first short-term goal of going with his sons to watch an important football match, and booked a relaxing weekend break with his wife. He completely resisted any further checking.

In addition, he and the therapist planned how he would deal with a new health scare or relapse using the method outlined in Chapter 8. Gordon began to feel a lot stronger, and over the next few weeks realised that he had got his life back. A year later he telephoned the therapist to say that he was really well and he and his wife were well and happy, and not only had they taken up sailing again (the long-term goal), but they had bought a new boat.

Tina was encouraged to continue to exercise regularly. She felt better for this, which she considered would not have been the case if she were terminally ill. She began to put on a bit of weight and found it easier to cope with work. She began to make some longer-term goals, exploring the possibility of getting a work permit for Australia. With time, it began to sink in that in fact she did not have HIV, but had been suffering with anxiety and some depression. She knew she was getting better when she was asked for a date by a man at the fitness club and really quite enjoyed the experience.

Common problems encountered in management

Some sexually transmitted infections may be carried for years before suspicion or detection, and often it is impossible to say precisely how long the condition has been harboured. This can be very disturbing for many patients who can find it very difficult to accept that they have been walking around carrying this infection, which has consequences for their health in the future and which they have possibly passed on or could potentially pass on to others. Not knowing who passed the infection to them in the first place can make some people feel violated and especially vulnerable. In these circumstances, it can help to consider the various alternatives, including that the person who did pass on the infection may well have been unaware that they had a problem in the same way that the patient was unaware of their problem for years.

Most sexually transmitted infections occur in younger people, and if untreated can have serious implications for fertility, which is obviously a huge underlying cause for concern in many patients. For example, a young woman who is diagnosed with chlamydia may have no idea how long she has had it, and even in the absence of clinically obvious pelvic inflammatory disease, there is a possibility it may have caused some low-grade but potentially serious fallopian tubal damage. There is no simple test to clarify whether or not she is fertile and, although the chances are that she will be OK, she needs to wait until she is trying to conceive and failing before the complex, lengthy and at times invasive investigations are undertaken. *In vitro* fertilisation and the huge progress in reproductive biology generally have greatly improved the prospects for infertile couples, but this is not without cost. Treatment is complex and not always successful, and is emotionally demanding. Fertility is a massive underlying fear for many patients in genitourinary medicine clinics and may be at the root of their health anxiety.

Fears about the possibility of having an STI can also have a devastating effect on sexual activity and performance. It is important to ask about this and be informed enough to give permission for your patient to resume a normal sex life.

Some patients who attend genitourinary clinics do so as a result of assault. Rape, abusive relationships and child sexual exploitation, as well as sex trafficking and prostitution, are relatively common, and they are routinely asked about in these clinical settings. Some of this abuse may have been recent, but some may have occurred in the past and only now come to light. Any history of trauma requires sensitive handling and may call for more specialist help, but empathic enquiry and acceptance as well as a willingness to talk about the problem, especially if this is the first time it has been divulged, is incredibly important. Victims of any kind of abuse often feel ashamed and partly responsible for letting the abuse happen, as abusers try to instil this into their victims to keep them from telling others. It takes immense courage to divulge information of this kind, and to have it legitimised by someone in authority who believes them is a crucial first step.

CHAPTER 16

Pain management

Pain is experienced in the brain. It is influenced not only by the nerve pathways from the skin and other structures, such as the spine (e.g. sciatica), but also from other parts of the brain, including the areas concerned with anxiety. There is abundant evidence that people who are anxious experience more pain than those who are calm, and treatments such as yoga and acupuncture probably affect these pathways more than the simple sensory ones. There are also cultural variations in the experience of pain.

Pain is a symptom, not a disease, and lends itself to a broad range of management approaches, most of which are not going to be discussed further here. Yet, where anxiety is a component, particularly when people are interpreting what pain might mean in terms of illness, the strategies described earlier in this handbook can be very helpful. In the traditional medical treatment of pain, relief of symptoms is achieved mainly by giving analgesics, such as aspirin and paracetamol, in the first instance, extending to much more powerful drugs, including opiates, when the pain becomes more intense. Much pain is short lived and relatively easily managed by this approach, but when it becomes chronic it is generally more difficult to explain, and it often becomes extraordinarily troublesome and distressing.

Many of the ways in which pain is treated medically have their limitations. Analgesics, however they are administered, nerve blocks, various surgical ablative procedures, and 'TENS' machines (which deliver small electrical pulses to the body via electrodes placed on the skin) are rarely completely successful, especially for chronic pain, and physicians prescribing them often do so with the caveat that they are of limited use or may only help some individuals. Many pain-relief remedies can be bought over the internet and sometimes offer more than they deliver.

The problem with many parts of medicine is that the role of specialist is to identify areas of pathology in which they have particular knowledge, but there is a danger that this knowledge can be used inappropriately to fit the experience of pain to their area of expertise. As Todd (1983) commented about one of the most common forms of investigated pain, usually called non-cardiac chest pain, 'bogus cardiac diseases have been diagnosed on an enormous scale, mainly because attention has been concentrated on the cardiac manifestations, while the patient was ignored'.

It is also important to realise that severe, apparently intractable pain can be a symptom of depression. Of course, having chronic pain can also be a very depressing experience, as can worrying about it all the time. But for a group of patients in whom depression is identified, treating it will relieve the pain.

Identifying health anxiety in chronic pain

Identifying the health anxiety that can accompany chronic pain allows another approach to management, quite apart from management of the pain itself, which is now carried out in extreme cases by special pain clinics. This process is done by questioning along the lines of: 'What does the pain mean for you? Do you think there is something more serious underlying the pain? Do you feel that it is more serious than other medical professionals appear to think?'. Keeping a diary can also be very useful here, as recording throughout the day the severity of the pain, its effects and how worried the person is at the time can throw light on any association between the pain and anxiety. The worries can then be explored using the techniques described in this handbook.

The use of pie charts to help in chronic pain management

Some patients have to deal with living with chronic pain and, although this is beyond the remit of this handbook, helping a patient look at the different ways pain can affect them and consider whether there are things that could help is a very useful process. Constructing a pie chart that encompasses all the different aspects of how the pain is managed and how it affects the patient's life can be illuminating. This would include pain management with drugs/other therapies, how it affects work, leisure, relationships, sleep, mood, managing everyday tasks, carers (if involved), and the financial considerations. These are listed, and the patient and therapist work together to establish how much of the pie can be attributed to each one. This gives a clear picture of how the pain affects the patient's life. They then consider together which of these various aspects the patient may be able to work on or change. The next stage is considering the nature of any such change and how it could be effected.

This can be followed up by the analogy of a bus journey, which symbolises the patient's life. People can get on or off the bus, except for one passenger, 'chronic pain'. The patient is asked who is currently driving the bus, the patient or the pain. They are then asked that taking into consideration the fact that 'chronic pain' seems to have to stay on the bus, where exactly should it be? It could be driving, sitting in the passenger area or placed in the luggage compartment, out of sight. Although this analogy seems too simple, it can be extraordinarily helpful for some patients. They can get a better picture of how the pain is affecting them and it can help them choose to re-evaluate their situation and begin to make changes that can give them more control.

CHAPTER 17

Conclusions

I hope this section of the book, illustrating the practical application of the principles of cognitive–behavioural therapy in patients in different medical contexts, is helpful. I have focused on clinical conditions I have seen myself, but my belief is that all clinics in general hospitals will have people with abnormal health anxiety attending frequently, and the aim of these chapters is to show that the general approach I have described can be modified and used in all these situations. In each of them it is very helpful to have some knowledge of the pathology of each of the physical disorders commonly encountered in the clinics concerned. So nurses in dermatology clinics may frequently come across people with skin lesions, spots or blemishes that are clearly not serious, but it helps enormously to know which lesions do indicate a physical intervention. Similarly, in orthopaedic clinics people with joint and back problems may misinterpret symptoms when having physiotherapy and infer serious consequences that are part of health anxiety rather than progression of disease. It also helps greatly if the patient has confidence with the therapist's knowledge of physical illness, so that when they explore the psychological aspects, these only appear to be an extension of this knowledge rather than a 'special mental health problem'. I have reminded people reading this book on many occassions in previous pages that worry over health is real and understandable, and when people engage in tackling the worry they are not having complex psychotherapy, they are just getting their symptoms back into proportion.

The recognition and simple interventions outlined can be applied by all health professionals – so please do not be inhibited and start helping people troubled by health anxiety now.

References

Altamura AC, Carta MG, Tacchini G, *et al* (1998) Prevalence of somatoform disorders in a psychiatric population: an Italian nationwide survey: Italian Collaborative Group on Somatoform Disorders. *European Archives of Psychiatry to Clinical Neuroscience*, **248**, 267–271.

Aydemir O, Ozmen E, Küey L, *et al* (1997) Psychiatric morbidity and depressive symptomatology in patients with permanent pacemakers. *Pacing Clinical Electrophysiology*, **20**, 1628–1632.

Barsky AJ, Klerman GL (1983) Overview: hypochondriasis, bodily complaints, and somatic styles. *American Journal of Psychiatry*, **140**, 273–283.

Barsky AJ, Wyshak G, Klerman GL, *et al* (1990) The prevalence of hypochondriasis in medical out-patients. *Social Psychiatry and Psychiatric Epidemiology*, **25**, 89–94.

Barsky AJ, Orav EJ, Bates DW (2005) Somatization increases medical utilization and costs independent of psychiatric and medical comorbidity. *Archives of General Psychiatry*, **62**, 903–910.

Beck AT, Emery G, Greenberg RL (1985) *Anxiety Disorders And Phobias: A Cognitive Perspective*. Basic Books.

Beck AT, Brown G, Epstein N, *et al* (1988) An inventory for measuring clinical anxiety – psychometric properties. *Journal of Consulting & Clinical Psychology*, **56**, 893–897.

Bombardier CH, Buchwald D (1996) Chronic fatigue, chronic fatigue syndrome, and fibromyalgia: disability and health-care use. *Medical Care*, **34**, 924–930.

Faravelli C, Salvatori S, Galassi F, *et al* (1997) Epidemiology of somatoform disorders: a community survey in Florence. *Social Psychiatry and Psychiatric Epidemiology*, **32**, 24–29.

Gatchel RJ, Mayer TG, Eddington A (2006) MMPI disability profile: the least known, most useful screen for psychopathology in chronic occupational spinal disorders. *Spine*, **31**, 2973–2978.

Gureje O, Ustun TB, Simon GE (1997) The syndrome of hypochondriasis: a cross-national study in primary care. *Psychological Medicine*, **27**, 1001–1010.

Kroenke K, Spitzer RL, deGruy FV 3rd, *et al* (1997) Multisomatoform disorder: an alternative to undifferentiated somatoform disorder for the somatizing patient in primary care. *Archives of General Psychiatry*, **54**, 352–358.

Lloyd AR, Pender H (1992) The economic impact of chronic fatigue syndrome. *Medical Journal of Australia*, **157**, 599–601.

Lucock MP, Morley S (1996) The Health Anxiety Questionnaire. *British Journal of Health Psychology*, **1**, 137–150.

Marcus DK, Hughes KT, Arnau RC (2008) Health anxiety, rumination, and negative affect: a mediational analysis. *Journal of Psychosomatic Research*, **64**, 495–501.

Mayou R, Kirmayer LJ, Simon G, *et al* (2005) Somatoform disorders: time for a new approach in DSM-V. *American Journal of Psychiatry*, **162**, 847–855.

Nimnuan C, Hotopf M, Wessely S (2001) Medically unexplained symptoms: an epidemiological study in seven specialities. *Journal of Psychosomatic Research*, **51**, 361–367.

Polatin PB, Kinney RK, Gatchel RJ, *et al* (1993) Psychiatric illness and chronic low-back pain. The mind and the spine–which goes first? *Spine*, **18**, 66–71.

Ruo B, Rumsfeld JS, Hlatky MA, *et al* (2003) Depressive symptoms and health-related quality of life: the heart and soul study. *JAMA*, **290**, 215–221.

Salkovskis PM (1989) Somatic problems. In *Cognitive Therapy for Psychiatric Problems: A Practical Guide* (eds H Hawton, PM Salkovskis, J Kirk, *et al*), pp. 235–276. Oxford University Press.

Salkovskis PM (1996) The cognitive approach to anxiety: threat beliefs, safety seeking behaviour, and the special case of health anxiety and obsessions. In *Frontiers of Cognitive Therapy: The State of the Art and Beyond*, pp. 48–74. Guilford Press.

Salkovskis PM, Clark DM (1993) Panic disorder and hypochondriasis. *Advances in Behaviour Research and Therapy*, **15**, 23–48.

Salkovskis PM, Warwick HM (1986) Morbid preoccupations, health anxiety and reassurance: a cognitive–behavioural approach to hypochondriasis. *Behaviour Research and Therapy*, **24**, 597–602.

Salkovskis PM, Clark DM, Gelder MG (1996) Cognition–behaviour links in the persistence of panic. *Behaviour Research and Therapy*, **34**, 453–458.

Salkovskis PM, Rimes KA, Warwick HMC, *et al* (2002) The Health Anxiety Inventory: development and validation of scales for the measurement of health anxiety and hypochondriasis. *Psychological Medicine*, **32**, 843–853.

Seivewright H, Salkovskis P, Green J, *et al* (2004) Prevalence and service implications of health anxiety in genitourinary medicine clinics. *International Journal of STD & AIDS*, **15**, 519–522.

Seivewright H, Green J, Salkovskis P, *et al* (2008) Cognitive–behavioural therapy for health anxiety in a genitourinary medicine clinic: randomised controlled trial. *British Journal of Psychiatry*, **193**, 332–337.

Tattersall R, Gregory R, Selby C, *et al* (1991) Course of brittle diabetes: 12-year follow-up. *BMJ*, **302**, 1240–1243.

Todd JW (1983) Query cardiac pain. *Lancet*, **362**, 330–332.

Tyrer PJ (1973) Relevance of bodily feelings in emotion. *Lancet*, **301**, 915–916.

Tyrer P, Lee I, Alexander J (1980) Awareness of cardiac function in anxious, phobic and hypochondriacal patients. *Psychological Medicine*, **10**, 171–174.

Tyrer P, Cooper S, Crawford M, *et al* (2011a) Prevalence of health anxiety problems in medical clinics. *Journal of Psychosomatic Research*, **71**, 392–394.

Tyrer H, Tyrer P, Lovett I (2011b) Adapted cognitive behaviour therapy for medically unexplained symptoms in secondary care reduces hospital contacts. *Psychosomatics*, **52**, 194–196.

Tyrer H, Ali L, Cooper F, *et al* (2013) The Schedule for Evaluating Persistent Symptoms (SEPS): a new method of recording medically unexplained symptoms. *International Journal of Social Psychiatry*, **59**, 281–287.

Warwick HM, Salkovskis PM (1990) Hypochondriasis. *Behaviour Research and Therapy*, **28**, 105–117.

Further reading

Asmundson GJG, Taylor S, Cox BJ (eds) (2001) *Health Anxiety: Clinical and Research Perspectives on Hypochondriasis and Related Conditions*. John Wiley & Sons.

Taylor S, Asmundson GJG (2004) *Treating Health Anxiety: A Cognitive Behavioral Approach*. Guilford Press.

Index

Compiled by Linda English

Printed in the United States
by Baker & Taylor Publisher Services